Building Resilience in Families Under Stress

Building Resilience in Families Under Stress

Supporting families affected by parental substance misuse and/or mental health problems

A handbook for practitioners

Second edition

Emma Sawyer and Sheryl Burton

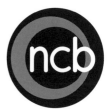

NCB's vision is a society in which all children and young people contribute, are valued and their rights are respected. NCB aims to:

- reduce inequalities of opportunity in childhood
- ensure children and young people can use their voice to improve their lives and the lives of those around them
- improve perceptions of children and young people
- enhance the health, learning, experiences and opportunities of children and young people
- encourage the building of positive and supportive relationships for children and young people with families, carers, friends and communities
- provide leadership through the use of evidence and research to improve policy and practice.

NCB has adopted and works within the UN Convention on the Rights of the Child.

Published by the NCB

NCB, 8 Wakley Street, London EC1V 7QE
Tel: 0207 843 6000
Website: www.ncb.org.uk
Registered charity number: 258825

NCB works in partnership with Children in Scotland (www.childreninscotland.org.uk) and Children in Wales (www.childreninwales.org.uk).

© National Children's Bureau 2012

ISBN: 978 1 907969 49 2

Second edition published 2012
First edition published 2009

British Library Cataloguing in Publication Data
A catalogue record for this book is available from the British Library

Typeset by Saxon Graphics Ltd, Derby, UK
Printed and bound by Hobbs the Printers, Totton, Hampshire, UK

Contents

List of practice examples

Preface to second edition

The current economic outlook is extremely challenging for those families already disadvantaged by poverty and social exclusion. For those also affected by parental mental health and/or substance misuse problems the outlook is bleaker still. Inflation and benefit changes have already taken a toll on family budgets, while unemployment looks set to continue on an upward trajectory for the foreseeable future. For those families with additional vulnerabilities, such as mental health and /or substance misuse problems these additional stressors are likely to compound and exacerbate existing difficulties. The consequences for children's welfare should families not receive the right support are likely to be severe.

People with mental health and substance misuse problems are already at increased likelihood of being in poverty or on low incomes. Additionally, while there are some signs of change in the attitudes of employers towards employing people with experience of mental illness, the problems of stigma and discrimination in the workplace are still major and these challenges are likely to increase as unemployment and insecurity about future job prospects rise.

Fear of being judged as 'not coping' or being a 'poor parent' can increase the tendency for families affected by parental mental health and/or substance misuse problems to withdraw and close in on themselves, increasing their social isolation. Contrary to what might be expected, given the persistent political rhetoric and apparent public support for protecting and supporting the vulnerable and disadvantaged, evidence suggests that attitudes towards those in need tend to harden during recession, further increasing the likelihood of exclusion and stigma. Thus, while services may be preserved for those in the greatest difficulty, the increased stigma associated with such services and the fear of being judged deter families affected by parental mental health/substance misuse problems from seeking help, with those already fearful of claiming services becoming even more reluctant to do so.

Within this context it is more imperative than ever that social workers and those with professional and agency responsibilities provide assistance to the most vulnerable, should work hard to decrease stigma, increase political and public understanding of the challenges facing families, and help to build the resilience of the families and children experiencing increased stress.

The notion of building resilience is particularly apt within the current context, given that central to the concept of resilience is the ability to withstand and even thrive despite experiencing significant life-adversities, for example poverty, parental mental health problems, domestic abuse, neglect. The concept of resilience offers a positive framework for working with the strengths of the child, family and wider community to boost resilience and effect positive change.

Building Resilience in Families Under Stress provides professionals with practical assistance in translating the concept into practice reality. It provides models, frameworks, examples and pointers to support them in their task of helping families affected by parental mental health and substance misuse problems so that they can better meet children's needs.

Sheryl Burton

Acknowledgements

We would like to thank The Parenting Fund for funding the Building Resilience project and the publication of the first edition of this handbook.

The first edition was written by Emma Sawyer, senior development officer at the National Children's Bureau (NCB), with assistance from Sheryl Burton, director, and Steve Howell, information development officer, Social Inclusion department, NCB. The second edition has been updated by Sheryl Burton with specific contributions from Zoe Renton, Head of Policy, NCB and Rhian Beynon, Head of Policy and Campaigns, Family Action, and with assistance fom Kate Thomas, Projects Assistant.

Thanks to all the original contributors of practice examples and to the agencies and professionals who participated in the Building Resilience project by attending workshops and sharing ideas, experiences and practice examples, including the following workshop speakers:

David Bailey, Amynta Cardwell, Donald Forrester, Tracey Hicks, Ellen Marks. Rose De Paeztron, Christine Puckering, Wendy Robinson, Catherine Shaw, Jo Tunnard, and Michele Wates.

Thanks to advisory group members for their time and expertise in the planning, development and undertaking of the project and contributing their ideas for this handbook:

Jo Tunnard (chair; and writer, researcher and consultant)
Debbie Cowley (director of practice development, Parenting UK)
Ruth Dalzell (freelance trainer and consultant)
Rose De Paeztron (head of strategic development, Family Welfare Association)
Dr Donald Forrester (reader in child welfare and director of the Child and Family Welfare Research Unit, Bedfordshire University)
Eva Geser (coordinator, Families and Prevention Programme, Adfam)
Brendan McLoughlin and Emma Raver (London Development Centre for Mental Health)
Suzanne Murray (parenting policy officer, Alcohol Concern)
Michele Wates (writer, researcher, campaigner)

The views expressed in the handbook are those of the authors and not necessarily those of all steering group members.

Introduction

This handbook emerged from the National Children's Bureau (NCB) project, Building Resilience and Supporting Relationships in Families under Stress, which ran from 2004 to 2006. The project's aim was to explore how relevant practitioners and professionals could support parenting more effectively in families affected by parental substance abuse or mental health problems, or both.

A number of agencies (see Appendix 1) were recruited to take part in the project, which involved attending a series of workshops. The workshops provided a rare opportunity to have a diverse group of practitioners and professionals come together – from adult, children and family services in the voluntary and statutory sectors – to consider and work on key issues. This process was interesting and informative for those involved and led to many participants developing and undertaking action plans locally to improve services.

The issues and points raised should be of interest and support to readers concerned with improving the support provided by agencies to families with multiple and complex difficulties.

Who is this handbook for?

The handbook is for practitioners and managers who are directly or indirectly involved in the provision of statutory or voluntary services to any family members affected by parental mental health problems; parental substance misuse or alcohol misuse; or a combination of these, who are working in:

- statutory and voluntary adult services, such as mental health or drug and alcohol teams
- statutory and voluntary children's services
- family-based services, such as children's or family centres, CAMHS, family group conferencing teams, parental mental health services
- universal services, such as health or education settings
- specialist services, such as drug treatment centres, psychiatric services or services aimed specifically at black and ethnic minority children and families
- any of the above services as commissioners or planners
- places other than the above but who have a professional, personal or academic interest in 'what helps' in supporting children and families in these circumstances.

How can it be used?

The handbook can be used by practitioners to help them consider the implications for children and families affected by parental substance misuse and mental health problems, how the negative impact of such circumstances can be minimised, and the interventions, support, knowledge or resources may be helpful. The handbook can be read cover to cover or dipped into whenever a section or practice example becomes particularly relevant. The practice examples are listed on page v.

What is in the handbook?

Chapter 1 provides some contextual information relating to parental substance misuse and mental health problems in families, including definitions; its prevalence; and the policy and legislative context. It ends with a brief discussion of current service responses in the UK for families in these circumstances.

Chapter 2 draws on literature and research to explore the potential impact on children and families of parental mental health problems and/or substance misuse, using the domains of the *Framework for the Assessment of Children in Need and their Families* (Department of Health 2000).

Chapter 3 explores the concept of resilience and highlights factors that can bolster families' ability to meet their children's needs and improve the life chances for young people in adverse circumstances.

Chapter 4 explores some of the barriers to the provision of effective support to families affected by parental substance misuse or parental mental health problems. Part One examines difficulties and barriers at the practice level and Part Two at the strategic and service planning level.

Chapter 5 considers 'What's needed' in order to make service responses more appropriate and supportive to families in these circumstances at the practice level.

Chapter 6 considers 'What's needed' at the strategic level of service planning.

The Further resources section provides information about relevant organisations and resources, which may assist in developing planning and practice.

The practice examples

The practice examples come from a range of sources; many describe approaches taken by agencies that participated in the Building Resilience project, while others were brought to the attention of participants or to the author throughout the life of the project. Not all of these examples are as 'best practice', as we have not been in a position to assess their effectiveness, but they do demonstrate useful ideas or potentially helpful approaches.

1. Context, legislation and policy

A large number of families are affected by parental substance misuse or parental mental health problems, or both. Apart from the direct effects upon the adults and children within those families, the indirect impact on the various relevant services working with them is 'pervasive, hidden and under recognised' (Kearney and others 2003). This chapter argues that most parents with these problems remain concerned for the welfare of their children and can cope with their parental responsibilities given adequate support. While asserting that the welfare of the child must always remain the paramount concern of professionals working with such families, it argues that there is often scope for professional responses to parental substance misuse and mental health issues to be more effective in supporting parents to safeguard the welfare of their children.

This chapter provides definitions of key terms and concepts used in this book; and statistics to indicate the numbers of children and families affected. It gives a broad outline of the policy and legislative context, highlighting the fact that policies and services are seldom coordinated and rarely take the necessary 'whole family approach' in interventions. The importance of the parenting role in many adult lives, and the likely impact of parental mental health/substance misuse problems on any children in such families, are too often overlooked by agencies whose primary focus is on the individual adult client.

Underpinning principles

Most parents, including those who have substance misuse and/or mental health difficulties, are deeply concerned for the welfare of their children. Many parents with substance misuse and/or mental health difficulties, given the right support, are nonetheless able to parent their children well. However, when parents lack the personal resources or external support required to meet their children's needs, their children suffer. It is therefore essential that practitioners – in all relevant fields – do not lose sight of children's needs and act in a timely and appropriate manner in order to meet them.

The interests of the child and their right to be protected from harm are always paramount. In addition to this, though, there is often much that can and should be done to support parenting and safeguard children. Such support can prevent parents' problems escalating to a point where the removal of the child from their parents' care becomes unavoidable. At all stages, it is worth professionals asking: *Given that this is the situation, what are the needs of this child? What are the immediate and longer term risks to this child? What things can be done that will minimise the impact of this on the child? And what might make a difference to how well the parents can meet or understand the needs and experiences of their child? Can these changes be achieved within a timeframe that will meet the child's needs?*

Central to the Building Resilience project and this handbook, is a belief that more often than not there is scope for practitioner responses to parental substance misuse and mental health problems to be more effective in supporting parenting and, in turn, the welfare of children.

Stigmatisation of such parents is a major factor in both worsening their circumstances and in reducing the likelihood of them feeling able to access or ask for support. An increased awareness of stigma and negative assumptions that can compound parents' difficulties can lead to more thorough, open explorations of their needs and potential.

Also, an increased understanding among relevant practitioners of what factors are likely to enhance the resilience of children and their families would enable them to respond more confidently and proactively to family difficulties.

This handbook then is about supporting families with substance misuse or mental health problems, or both, and enabling parents and their children to cope better with their circumstances. It explores and shares information that might help practitioners to harness the motivation, strengths and values of many adults. There can obviously be times when there is a tension between the needs of children and the priorities and capacities of their parents. In these circumstances it will sometimes, regrettably, be necessary for children to be removed from the care of their parents. However, this need can be averted in some cases if professional knowledge and skills are enhanced to enable services to work more preventively and proactively with parents. Early intervention and support to families can be effective in keeping them together, safeguarding children and helping parents to support their child's well-being.

Definitions

Resilience

> *a universal capacity which allows a person, group or community to prevent, minimise or overcome the damaging effects of adversity*

> (Grotberg 1997, p.7 in Newman and Blackburn 2002)

Certain factors (often referred to as 'protective factors'), such as the presence of an unconditionally supportive adult from either within the family or external to it, have been seen in a number of studies to play an important part in minimising the impact of family problems on children. The presence of such factors can be seen as leading to better outcomes for children. Resilience factors are discussed further in Chapter 3.

Mental health problems

This handbook focuses specifically on circumstances where parents or their children are experiencing problems and these are linked to mental health. This will include minor mental health problems, such as a one-off or occasional period of depression or anxiety, through to the most severe disorders, such as bipolar disorder or schizophrenia. However, minor problems are only included if it can be said of the parents experiencing them that they are:

> *experiencing such emotional distress that they find it hard to function as well as they would wish, and they and/or others are concerned about the actual or likely impact this is having on their children*

> (Tunnard 2004, p.7)

Some studies referred to within this handbook may use the term 'mental illness' instead. Where this is used, the following definition may be useful:

A term used by doctors and other health professionals to describe clinically recognisable patterns of psychological symptoms or behaviour causing acute or chronic ill-health, personal distress or distress to others

(World Health Organisation 1992)

For definitions of specific categories of mental health diagnoses, Falkov (1998, pp. 37–55) provides summaries; and some of the mental health related websites listed in the Further resources section of this handbook provide useful information.

Substance misuse

This term includes those using any substances, including alcohol, prescribed medication or illegal drugs. 'Misuse' rather than 'use' is referred to in order to distinguish between the recreational user and the dependent user whose behaviour, mood or other life circumstances are adversely affected by their use of the substance.

Another term that is often used in this handbook, particularly if referring to information from the *Hidden Harm* report from the Advisory Council on the Misuse of Drugs (Gruer and Ainsworth 2003), is **problem drug use**. The Advisory Council defines problem drug use as that which has:

serious negative consequences of a physical, psychological, social and interpersonal, financial or legal nature for users and those around them

Whilst much of the discussion about parental substance misuse will be general, occasionally alcohol misuse is referred to separately because it brings with it some distinct issues. Also, services are often set up separately for drug users and alcohol users within voluntary and statutory services.

For the classification of individual drugs and their effects, there are a number of useful summaries: FRANK (www.talktofrank.com), Kroll and Taylor (2003), and Hart and Powell (2006).

Dual diagnosis

This is a term used to describe the presence in an individual of two or more categories of need from a range including, for example, learning disabilities, mental health issues and substance misuse issues. Where the term is used in this handbook, unless specified otherwise, it is to indicate the presence of mental health problems along with substance misuse issues.

Defining dual diagnosis can be contentious. Miller (1994) defines it thus:

The strict definition of dual diagnosis means that another disorder exists independent of an addictive disorder. The key words are 'another' and 'independent'

(Miller, NS (ed) 1994)

Using the definition above raises the question as to how 'independent' substance misuse and mental health problems are from each other. For example, in some circumstances it can be argued that substance use has led to mental health difficulties or, conversely, that substance use is a form of 'self-medication' for emotional distress arising from mental health problems. Therefore an understanding of the mental health issues *and* the substance use, in addition to a consideration of the interaction between the two, is necessary.

A high number of adults have both mental health and substance misuse difficulties. Morris and Wates (2006) report on studies that found such overlaps within groups of services' users. For example, one study found 75 per cent of drug service users and 85 per cent of alcohol service users had additional mental health problems; and 44 per cent of Community Mental Health Team users reported substance misuse or problem drinking within the previous 12 months.

Velleman (2004), Falkov (1998) and Cleaver and others (1999) found dual diagnosis to be associated with reduced treatment compliance; more severe mental health problems; greater risks of self-harm and harm to others; greater family discord; an increased likelihood of domestic violence; and increased social and financial difficulties.

Whilst the presence of the two issues together cause an increased professional concern (Forrester 2000), which is potentially compounded by services tending not to be geared up to meeting overlapping needs effectively, the interrelatedness of the mental health and substance use are not explored in detail in this handbook.

Prevalence

Mental health problems and substance misuse are not readily measurable in terms of prevalence. Much of people's emotion and behaviour is unknowable and it is only when people are formally diagnosed or identified through services that individuals are included within prevalence figures. Secrecy – and the inevitability of this due to stigma and illegality (in the case of drug use) – further limits the chances of prevalence figures being accurate. It is likely therefore that the figures used by official bodies, such as the Advisory Council on the Misuse of Drugs, are underestimations. Also mental health varies over time, with many people experiencing episodes of problems but feeling well in between. Similarly, substance use or misuse is a behaviour and even those who view addiction as a permanent illness that has to be managed would acknowledge that its impact, visibility and how it is seen and experienced by individuals changes over time. That said, the following figures that are available give some indication of prevalence.

Mental health problems

One in six adults experience at least one period of minor mental health difficulty, such as depression or anxiety, in their lifetimes (Singleton and others 2004). Prevalence is highest in women and lone parents (Meltzer and others 1995) and those in socially disadvantaged groups or communities. One in forty adults experience serious and enduring mental health problems in their lifetime, such as schizophrenia, severe depression, bipolar disorder or dual diagnosis (Tunnard 2004).

At least a quarter of adults known to mental health services are parents; a third of children known to adolescent mental health services have parents with a psychiatric disorder; and parental mental health or substance misuse is recorded in at least a third of families referred to social services due to child protection concerns (Falkov 1998).

Alcohol misuse

Children known to be living with parental alcohol misuse are thought to number between 780,000 and 1.3 million (Prime Minister's Strategy Unit 2003), which equates to one in 11 children living with problem drinkers (Turning Point 2006). Men are more likely to report hazardous drinking and signs of dependence than women (Office for National Statistics in Gopfert and others 2004) and there has been a growth in problem drinking overall since the early 1990s.

Drug misuse

The number of adults known to have 'problem drug use' (as defined by the Advisory Council on the Misuse of Drugs) is growing; and the annual numbers of those accessing drug services doubled between 1996 and 2000. Conservative estimates are that between 200,000 and 300,000 children in England and Wales are affected by parental problem drug use.

Legislation and policy context

The legislative and policy background to service provision for families affected by parental mental health, substance misuse and child welfare issues is complex, with a raft of legal and policy measures that have been introduced at different times and for different reasons. The consequence of this can be a lack of clarity and a failure by legislators and service planners to make links between them.

It can be difficult to keep abreast of the policy and legislative context within one professional arena, for example within children's social care or adult mental health. It is all the more difficult to keep up with policy or legislation that colleagues in other fields work. The following areas of policy and legislation (though not exhaustive) are of particular relevance:

- children's and adult social care
- community care
- mental health
- drugs and alcohol
- families and parenting
- welfare reform
- disability equality/anti-discrimination.

A summary of the above areas of policy and legislation (which highlights issues relevant to parenting and family welfare) can be found in Appendix 2.

On the whole, legislation and policies that relate to mental health and to drugs have tended to focus on the single adult user. They have not placed sufficient responsibilities and duties on the responding services to meet wider families' needs. In fact they have often failed to acknowledge any overlap or tension between the rights and responsibilities of one member of the family (for example, a parent) with those of another (for example a child or young carer). The 1995 10-year Drug Strategy (Home Office, Department of Health and Department for Education 1995), for example, focused on adult drug use as a criminal activity and did not acknowledge parenting as a feature of many drug users' lives and responsibilities. There was a tendency to focus on the consequences of parental drug use rather than on helping parents manage or change their use of drugs. The 2008 strategy (HM Government 2008) attempted to redress this, paying much more attention to supporting drug users as parents. More recently, the coalition government revised Drug Strategy (HM Government 2010) places an emphasis on preventing problems from arising, stresses the need for adult and children's services to devise protocols for working together and states that drug and alcohol services should be represented on Local Safeguarding Children's Boards (LSCBs).

Whilst much of the legislation and policy aimed at children does broadly include addressing their needs in relation to any familial factors affecting them, the implementation of such policies tends to be seen as the domain of children's services and not (in practice) those whose primary clients are adults.

The Children Act 2004 provides the legislative framework for the previous government's Every Child Matters agenda, which sought to strengthen partnership working across agencies to promote children's well-being. While the coalition government has removed requirements to establish a Children's Trust Board and prepare a Local Authority Children and Young People's Plan, many of the provisions of the Children Act 2004 remain in place. This includes:

- a reciprocal duty among a list of partners to promote cooperation to improve the well-being of children (section 10)
- a duty on partners to safeguard and promote the welfare of children.

Whilst the separation of adults and children's services have been largely supported through legislation, there has been recognition in guidance and policy of the importance of bridging these divides. *Guidance on the Statutory Chief Officer Post of the Director of Adult Social Services* and the *Best Practice Guidance on the Role of the Director of Adult Social Services* (Department of Health 2006) as well as the *Statutory Guidance on the Roles and Responsibilities of the Director of Children's Services* and *Lead Member for Children's Services* (DfES 2005a) looked at the links that should be made between adult and children's social services and, in particular, the complementary roles of the Director of Adult Social Services (DASS) and the Director of Children's Services (DCS). The needs of families are recognised, and the best practice guidance recommends establishing clear protocols between adult and children's services; and making sure that procedures for joint working are in place to ensure that the needs of the child are considered when a social worker is assessing the needs of, or providing a service to, the parent.

To conclude, although the legislation and policy does not consistently acknowledge 'parenting' and the links between children and adults (in relation to services, needs, rights and responsibilities), there are some provisions within the legislation and some drivers towards addressing this. There are a number of similarities in the issues facing services, including the tension between high eligibility thresholds and the vision of providing preventative services. The current drive towards more joint commissioning, a greater 'outcomes focus', needs analysis and more multi-agency working, is positive. However, it is essential that at a local level, opportunities are not lost for adults and children's services to link in with each other in the development of these changes to services.

> in a system that 'thinks family' contact with any service offers an open door into a broader system of joined up support ... Front-line staff are alert to wider individual and family risk factors, and practitioners consider the causes and wider impacts of presenting problems.
>
> (Social Exclusion Task Force 2008 *Think Family: Improving the life chances of families at risk*)
> http://www.cabinetoffice.gov.uk/social_exclusion_task_force/families_at_risk/

The service context

The impact of both parental mental health issues and substance misuse on the work of relevant services is 'pervasive, hidden and under recognised' (Kearney and others 2003), with a lack of information systems in place to capture the size of the problem. In 1997, NISW (National Institute for Social Work) carried out interviews with social workers in child care teams who estimated that 50 to 90 per cent of the parents on their caseloads were affected by mental health issues, substance misuse or alcohol misuse. Despite the lack of official statistics on parental mental health issues, it has been estimated that up to 30 per cent of the adults in contact with specialised mental health services have dependent children (Melzer 2008). According to the same Family Welfare Association briefing paper, *Families Affected by Parental Mental Health Difficulties*, unpublished data supplied by the Department of Work and Pensions suggested that, at May 2005, there were 198,000 parents receiving incapacity benefit who had a mental and behavioural disorder.

The organisation of services aimed at supporting such families (or the individuals within them) is complicated and disparate. A complex range of advice, assessment and treatment services are available to varying extents in local areas. Services struggle to work together in a coordinated way. Problems for families in accessing appropriate support are therefore common. Resource constraints (and the resulting high eligibility thresholds) within health and social care services mean tight gatekeeping and responses that tend to be reactive and crisis-led.

The Department for Education (DfE, formerly DCSF) wants those who most need parental and family support to be able to access well-coordinated, high quality support early enough so as to reduce the number of vulnerable families who go on to develop complex problems in the future. The department's earlier analysis (DfES 2006a) confirming a gap between this desired state and the market still stands. It highlighted a focus by the statutory sector on remedial interventions with minimal resources for prevention; and suggested that this makes it unlikely that ongoing support is available for as long as parents need it, and that fathers and black and minority ethnic groups in particular are not being engaged with effectively, especially at the lower tiers of need.

Although Family Intervention projects have proven effective in tackling the needs of families in challenging circumstances, there are still too few services aimed at whole families and a lack of a joined-up approach between adults' and children's teams. There is also much evidence to show that, within adult social care provision, disabled parents (including parents with significant mental health support needs) are not having their needs in relation to their parenting role routinely assessed. This is despite the *Fair Access to Care Services* guidance (DH 2003a) being clear that they should be (DH and Social Services Inspectorate 2000, Wates 2002). There is only a very small number of drug agencies or adult mental health services aimed at additionally addressing the needs of children in these circumstances. A lack of supportive family-focused services is both failing to prevent poor outcomes and compounding them. While the coalition government's announcement of £450M to tackle the difficulties posed by those branded the most 'troubled' 120,000 families, is generally welcome, the effectiveness of the strategy is seen as significantly hampered because it is argued this covers only 40 per cent of the estimated cost at a time when statutory and voluntary sector services are under significant financial strain, with non-acute services already being pared back or lost.

Parental substance misuse

The outcomes for children in families where there is parental 'problem drug use' are known to be poor, with less than half of all problem drug-using parents in the UK living with their children (Gruer and Ainsworth 2003). Mostly, their children end up living with other relatives and 9 per cent become Looked After under the Children Act 1989.

In their research into parental substance misuse and child welfare in social services, Forrester and Harwin (2006) found a third of cases in overall social work case-loads (in four London boroughs) had substance misuse issues noted. Of this sample, 36 per cent involved crack cocaine use, although the most concerning substance use (in numbers and in impact) was alcohol misuse. They found, despite substance use being so prevalent among case-loads, that social workers were poorly prepared for working with these issues. Two years after they first looked at case files:

- 54 per cent of the children no longer lived at home
- a third had been removed by care proceedings
- the majority lived with kinship carers, with or without a court order attached
- 8 per cent were adopted
- 16 per cent were in short-term foster care.

Hart and Powell (2006) also found, in their work with two local authorities, that less than half the children that were being worked with who had drug-misusing parents were living at home and that prospects for their return were poor. The children of drug-misusing parents accounted for:

- 18.5 per cent of the looked after children population
- 20 per cent of children on the child protection registers (this was not including children of alcohol-misusing parents).

Overall, Forrester and Harwin's (2006) research pointed to under-intervention in relation to violence in the home and in relation to alcohol use (particularly when these occurred together). If children in such families were removed from home this happened much later, when they were older, even though in the sample the overall outcomes were worse for those who remained at home. Velleman (2004) similarly found that drug-misusing parents were more likely to be rated high risk and to have their children removed than alcohol-misusing parents. This could be in part due to a higher level of familiarity by workers with alcohol; the illegality or stigmatisation of substance misuse; and a lack of recognition of the potential long-term impact on children of exposure to parental alcohol misuse.

It seems that whilst intervention is occurring, it is occurring at the 'heavy end' of family difficulty – too late and with the child protection process and legal intervention all too often being seen as the only realistic response by that stage. For children of alcohol-misusing parents, intervention is occurring even later. A lack of preventative services seems to be linked to high eligibility criteria; a lack of understanding about how to intervene constructively with families; and a reluctance by families to ask for help for fear their children will be removed.

Mental health problems

The picture is similarly bleak in relation to responses to parental mental health difficulty. Thresholds for intervention and in particular for specialist services are so high that they are not accessible for families assessed as having anything less than 'severe' or 'acute' need (Tunnard 2004). It is very difficult for families with mild or moderate mental health issues to access preventative support (from statutory services) in relation to their mental health needs, even though the impact on their children could be felt to be 'severe'.

As far as possible, services aim to support adults with mental health problems to remain in the home with support, but this can only be beneficial if the interrelated needs of other family members in the home are considered appropriately. (See Practice example for how Tower Hamlets' Home Treatment Team is addressing these issues.)

Tunnard (2004) reported that there was a lack of appropriate services provided to parents with mental health difficulties; with a significant number receiving no outside help. Of those that did receive help, many found it intrusive and of poor quality. Alarming problems were found in particular with home support services.

When it is necessary for parents with mental health problems to be hospitalised, this can be traumatic for them and their family members. Psychiatric wards can be potentially frightening places for children and do not provide privacy or a suitable environment for parents and their children to have positive contact. There is a lack of family-friendly facilities, although there are some examples of family rooms being set up, such as the one at Stoddart House in Aintree (arising from Barnardo's Keeping the Family in Mind project collaboration with Mersey Care. See the *Training and development resources* section in the Further resources section). But these are the exceptions rather than the rule.

Also, as a result of resource constraints mental health care is often inadequate, both within the community and for inpatients. For example, while access to some approaches such as cognitive behavioural therapy is helping some service users, overall access to talking therapies is lacking due to long waiting lists, financial constraints and a lack of therapists.

2. The potential impact on children and families

This chapter gives an overview of key research findings on the risks and impacts of parental substance misuse and mental health problems on children. Findings indicate that these parental problems are usually of great significance to their children. Possible adverse impacts are outlined in terms of the three domains of the *Framework for the Assessment of Children in Need and their Families: Family and environmental factors, parenting capacity and children's developmental needs* (Department of Health 2000).

This chapter stresses that assessing such impacts on individual children and families requires analysis, reflection and self-awareness in those undertaking it. A clear focus on questioning and exploring the everyday experience of family members is needed – rather than placing an overemphasis on crisis or 'unusual' incidents – along with a child-focused ecological approach, and knowledge of research and other evidence about effective interventions.

This chapter provides an essential overview of some of the research available on the potential implications for children and families when parental substance misuse or parental mental health problems are present, to increase the awareness that relevant practitioners and professionals have of these issues. This awareness should be utilised in tandem with an understanding of resilience factors (discussed in Chapter 3) and approaches to support (discussed in Chapter 5) that might help alleviate or reduce negative impacts.

Parents who misuse substances, and those with mental health difficulties, are obviously not homogeneous groups and there will be significant diversity of experience. However, from what is known, it is evident that parental substance misuse and parental mental health problems are usually of great significance to the welfare of families. Literature and research relating to parenting in these circumstances have pointed to a range of common issues, such as experiences of stigma and discrimination; poverty; isolation; a potential inconsistency of care; and disruptions and crises.

It is important to be aware that in the majority of the literature and research (particularly relating to parental mental health), 'parent' is often synonymous with 'mothers', with less consideration given to fathers and the impact on their relationship with their children. And most of the information that is drawn on focuses on identifying risks and poor outcomes that are often associated with such parental difficulties, rather than focusing on 'what goes well'. As the majority of studies are based on samples of parents who are known to services, the findings are skewed (Olsen and Wates 2003). There has been little research on the impact of support, that is on how parents and children fare when families are given appropriate and timely support. That said, the information that is available is useful if viewed in context and applied critically with a focus towards families' individual circumstances.

Impact of parental mental health problems

Whilst most parents with mental health difficulties don't pose a risk of child abuse to their children, risks are heightened if their difficulties are psychotic in nature or are coupled with substance misuse. An increased risk of maltreatment by mothers with severe depression and those with schizophrenia who draw their children into their negative delusions has also been long established (Falkov 1998). Even where parents don't pose a physical risk to their children, there is a possibility of children being frightened by severe mood changes or bizarre or unusual behaviours when their parents are unwell. In all cases, the risk of difficulties escalating and the levels of unmet need or risk increasing are compounded by a lack of appropriate responses from services.

For additional information see the useful overviews of research that have been done by Cleaver and others (1999), Tunnard (2002a, 2002b and 2004) and Kroll and Taylor (2003), and which are drawn on in this summary.

Below is an exploration of some of the issues known to be frequently associated with these circumstances. The three domains of the *Framework for the Assessment of Children in Need and their Families* (Department of Health 2000) and of the *Common Assessment Framework* (HM Government 2006b) – Family and environmental factors, Parenting capacity and Child's developmental needs – have been used as headings for ease of reference. For those who are not familiar with the three domains they are based on the Assessment triangle (Figure 1), which forms the basis for initial and core assessments undertaken by children and family social workers in conjunction with other relevant practitioners and professionals. This 'ecological' approach is based on the premise that the well-being of a family can best be understood if there is an appreciation of the ways in which the children's developmental needs, parents' capacity to respond to those needs, and wider environmental factors interact with one another over time (NSPCC 2000).

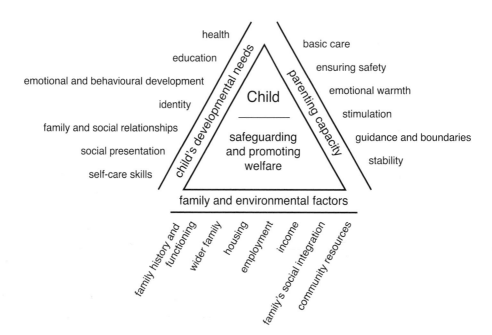

Figure 1: Assessment triangle

Family and environmental factors

Anecdotal evidence and inspections have highlighted that 'family and environmental factors' is often the 'missing side of the triangle' within assessments (Jack and Gill 2003) because not enough attention is paid to considering the wider social and environmental factors that affect families and, in turn, parenting. One reason could be that factors such as poverty and deprivation are hard to influence at the practitioner or indeed local services level. Such issues therefore come to be seen as too difficult, residual or less relevant to the 'task' of assessing needs of individual children and families. However, understanding and acknowledging the context of a family's experience is essential to good assessment practice, and service users are likely to be more engaged with services when their whole experience is recognised and attention is paid to the challenges they genuinely face in their lives, which originate both within their internal and external world (Kroll and Taylor 2003).

Family history and functioning

Previous experience of parents

Many adults with substance misuse and/or mental health problems have experienced adversity in their own childhoods. Exploring parents' experiences of being parented, along with establishing how family members experience each other in the present day, can lead to useful insights. Mental health issues may well be triggered by previous experiences or exacerbated by the ways in which the family functions in the present day (such as a culture of secrecy or 'not complaining') and substance misuse may be a way of avoiding or being distracted from other problems (Bennett 1989).

Support of partner

Where only one parent has mental health problems or substance misuse issues, their partner can play a key role in minimising the negative impact on children. In relation to substance misuse, studies have highlighted the benefit to children of stable relationships.

Where mothers have agreed that they wanted and planned to reduce their substance use, their partner's support of that decision was 'the most effective influence for positive change'. However, a partner's own substance use was cited as the most negative influence (Tunnard 2002a). Much of the research about this is specific to mothers with mental health or substance misuse issues, although it seems likely to apply to both sexes.

'Partner difficulties' have been found to be a common and contributory source of stress to parents with mental health problems who are in touch with statutory services and this is especially the case for depressed mothers (Tunnard 2004).

Separations and changes

Children are at an increased likelihood of experiencing separations, which may be short or long term, including, for example, planned or emergency hospitalisation or treatment for parents. Sometimes separations are a result of children being removed from their parents' care for periods of respite in order to prevent or address a crisis situation in which the child or parent's needs would be compromised if they remained at home.

Children may experience a number of minor or major changes in their family, including in the roles that family members take on. For example, a 'well parent' may perform tasks and essentially step into the role normally held by the parent with mental health problems (Falkov 1998). Such changes can be unsettling and sometimes resisted by children.

Family conflict

Marital breakdown and parental tension are at increased risk of occurring in families where there is substance misuse or mental illness (Weissman and Paykel 1974). Unfortunately there are also significant associations between both mental health problems and substance misuse and domestic violence. Excessive alcohol use is also frequently associated with violence in families. Hamilton and Collins (1981) and Powers (1986) found 80 per cent of spouse-to-spouse violence to be alcohol related. It is difficult to untangle the interrelationship between substance use, mental health and family discord or violence. Hester and others (2003) stress that substance use can be seen in some cases as a response to domestic violence; and a consideration of such issues is important within assessments and dialogues with those affected.

Where conflict and domestic violence occur, outcomes for children worsen noticeably (Velleman 1993). If arguments involve the child (in reality or in the child's perception) the negative impact on children is increased further.

Wider family

Given the potential for separations, change and parental conflict, the role of other relatives is significant and extended family members often provide considerable support. However, parents with mental health problems can experience difficulties in maintaining positive relationships with wider family members; often due to stigma and when their behaviour results in disapproval or misunderstandings. Where the support of wider family or friends is available to families under stress, this is valued and becomes most crucial in times of crisis. Relatives are likely to need support and information to help them understand the needs and issues facing the parent (Tunnard 2004).

In the case of substance-misusing mothers, many report positive relationships with their mother or another female relative (Tunnard 2002a). However, in some cases, relationships with relatives may have broken down previously, due to the rejection of the parent because of their substance misuse or the secrecy surrounding it (Kroll and Taylor 2003), and in such instances proves a significant barrier to familial support being provided by the wider family.

Housing

There are higher rates of depression among the populations of deprived areas than in more affluent areas. Unsafe neighbourhoods, poor housing, overcrowding and disputes with neighbours all increase stress significantly and are more commonly experienced by depressed mothers than other mothers (Tunnard 2004). This is compounded further for black and minority ethnic families who additionally often experience racism and discrimination (Social Exclusion Unit 2004) within local areas.

For families affected by substance misuse, in many cases the financial demands of securing drugs on a daily basis can lead to a lack of furniture, and unpaid bills resulting in erratic supplies of utilities such as gas, electricity and telephone access. Sometimes failures to pay rent or mortgages lead to eviction and a succession of short-term unsuitable housing (Cleaver and others 1999).

Employment

The Social Exclusion Unit in its report highlights the tendency for adults with mental health problems to experience discrimination by potential employers; and for black and minority ethnic adults to experience additional discrimination on the grounds of both their health status and ethnicity when seeking work (Social Exclusion Unit 2004).

The unpredictable and inconsistent effect of drug or alcohol use on individuals can make it hard to sustain employment; Velleman (1993) found half of people treated for alcohol problems lost their jobs as a direct result of their drinking.

Income

People with mental health problems or substance misuse issues are at increased likelihood of being affected by poverty and to have low incomes. Sustained use, for example, of heroin or cocaine can be very expensive and diminish family resources. The link between poverty and drug use is complex but, overall, drug users tend to be found in higher numbers in socially deprived areas. People with mental health problems tend to be on low incomes (exacerbated by employment issues). This creates stress and in turn often compounds mental health problems as well as increasing the risk of substance misuse and relapse (Fraser and others 2006).

Family's social integration

There is increased likelihood of children in these circumstances experiencing isolation from a wider network of social support. This is in part due to the stigma and secrecy that often surround mental health and substance misuse issues, in addition to the social exclusion that results from poverty and deprivation. These difficulties are compounded further for some groups such as lone parent families and for black and minority ethnic families.

Isolated parents have fewer opportunities to get support from other parents; and their children are less likely to have friends visit them at home. Whilst Velleman and Orford (1999) did not find such isolation in problem-drinking families, they did find a knock-on effect on children's friendships. Often they were embarrassed by their homes and had a sense of 'being apart' from others.

When there is parental substance misuse, in some cases friends of the parent/family offer considerable support, whereas in others, friends and associates who are also involved in substance misuse can pose additional risks that are 'sometimes as difficult to control as the drug use itself' (Tunnard 2002a).

Community resources

A tendency for families to 'close in on themselves' due to social isolation is exacerbated by poor or stigmatising community resources and a fear of being judged as not coping or being a poor parent. With substance misuse this can result in families retreating further into a substance-using environment to the exclusion of wider support (Velleman 1993). This worsens further when there are specific cultural issues and increased stigma regarding drug or alcohol use (Patel 2000, Tunnard 2002a). Where families are affected by mental health issues, a tendency towards increased isolation due to stigma, poverty or wariness of services and of others, significantly increase vulnerability.

The availability of good community resources is an important factor affecting the level of adverse impact on families (Kroll and Taylor 2003). High quality and accessible childcare, health care, transport, leisure and educational facilities can all make a big difference to how isolated or supported families are.

Community resources that provide a range of services within one location can be particularly useful. For pregnant drug users for example, uptake of appointments within clinics is likely to be improved by the provision of accessible, multidisciplinary support in one location, given the often-chaotic lifestyles associated with drug use and the other barriers caused by social deprivation.

Parenting capacity

It is important to reiterate that many people with mental health difficulties and/or who use drugs do manage to care adequately for their children. However, many experience difficulties at some time or other in managing to meet their children's needs. If those with difficulties are insufficiently supported or the difficulties are too severe, it can result in children being 'in need', including being 'in need of protection'.

Basic care

In parents affected by mental health problems or substance misuse a lack of energy, alertness or motivation can – and often does – affect the likelihood of basic care and chores being performed consistently. This can affect activities such as maintaining bath and bedtime routines, regular mealtimes, household chores and hygiene, and getting children to school on time.

Deficits in children's care may be deemed individually as low-level concerns. But over time, neglect of children's physical care needs can be chronic and their impact enduring, not least if their health is affected or their hygiene, which can impact on self-esteem and relationships with others.

Ensuring safety

Substance misuse can lead to drowsiness and lack of physical coordination, increasing the risk of parental accidents, including dropping a baby or child, decreased awareness of environmental risks and lower levels of supervision, which can lead to accidents for children. Storing methadone (or other drugs) where children can access them can cause immediate and serious dangers to children.

The preoccupation that can come with dependence and withdrawal, due to drug use, is likely to lead to a poorer awareness of children's needs and a reduced sensitivity to risk (Bates and others 1999). Similarly, mental health problems, depression or intrusive thoughts, and the effects of medication may reduce awareness of risks to children.

Emotional warmth

Parents can exhibit 'emotional unavailability' at particular times, for example when they are particularly unwell, preoccupied, on medication, or using or withdrawing from drugs or alcohol. This can adversely affect children's identity, self-esteem and attachments.

'Low warmth' and 'high criticism' environments are associated with poorer outcomes for children. Such environments are prevalent where there is parental alcohol misuse and some problem drug use (Kroll and Taylor 2003, Brisby and others 1997), including amphetamine use, which can be associated with parental irritability and aggression (Tunnard 2002a).

Stimulation

Around 10 to 15 per cent of women are affected by a heightened risk of depression after childbirth (Falkov 1998) and are likely to spend less time touching and looking at their baby. Where postnatal depression or maternal depression continues, a lower quality of interaction is found in the child's second year and insecure attachment is more likely to become apparent in the child's third year (Tunnard 2004).

More generally, when parents become emotionally less available to their children (as a result of low mood, effects of medication or substance misuse, or due to substance withdrawal) this can result in a lack of stimulation and, in turn, disrupted attachments.

Guidance and boundaries

In the case of parental mental ill health, the effects of medication or the 'absent mindedness' or internal preoccupation that can accompany distress or depression can reduce parents' ability to supervise or set boundaries for their children. Conversely, parents experiencing delusions, paranoia or anxiety may be excessively concerned about real or imagined risks to their child, causing them to set over-rigid boundaries or to restrict freedom or opportunities for their child.

As children become older, the problems arising from a lack of consistency, for example behavioural problems, can become more pronounced.

Brisby and others (1997) found there was often an authoritarian parenting style in problem-drinking families, but that periods of inebriation can lead at other times to a more lax approach and indifference, which can be confusing and create unclear boundaries and insecurity for children.

Stability

Unpredictability within daily life is a feature for many children with parents with either mental health or substance misuse issues. In the case of substance misuse, if a parent's moods and the events of the day are dependent on whether and how they secure and take drugs, the child's world must seem a very unstable one. There is likely to be a lack of routine, structure and consistency, all of which are important factors for children's sense of security, confidence and boundaries. Planned family occasions or events may not happen and can be 'fraught with uncertainty' (Brisby and others 1997). For children this can lead to disappointment or a lack of positive experiences to draw from or look forward to. Rituals, defined by Velleman (2004, p.186) as 'repeated gathering or set modes of behaviour which define the occasion or the day as being special', are intended to cement family relationships. Alcohol or drug use can cause disruption to such occasions as this (Bennet and others 1987) as can parental mental health difficulties.

Children's developmental needs

Health

In families affected by parental substance misuse, the knock-on effects of poverty, poor diet, potential neglect and poor hygiene can have an adverse impact on children's health. This can be compounded if money that would otherwise be spent on children is diverted to drugs. Children of substance-misusing parents may also exhibit psychosomatic responses to anxiety such as headaches, bedwetting and stomach aches (Kroll and Taylor 2003). Also some health problems may not be picked up by school medical services due to absenteeism (Cleaver and others 1999). Young people whose parents misuse drugs are at increased risk of developing their own substance problems, which in turn adversely impact on their health. Overall, there is a lack of longitudinal studies regarding the impact of substance-misusing parents on the emotional and mental health of children and young people.

In her overview of mental health research, Tunnard (2004) reported that in the UK, children whose parents screened positive on a mental health questionnaire were three times more likely than others to have mental health problems themselves. As with substance misuse, there is a lack of longitudinal data in the UK concerning the impact of parental mental health problems on children's health. Some qualitative studies show children and young people of parents with mental health problems to be likely to experience increased anxiety, depression, and fear of not being able to cope with life; and physical symptoms such as asthma, epilepsy, hair and weight loss. The increased mental health risk could be due to genetic factors; feeling isolated or rejected as a child (including by the well parent if their attention was more focused on the unwell parent than the child); or learnt behaviour.

Education

The effect on routines and daily life of parental substance misuse or mental health problems can lead to erratic school attendance or difficulties with punctuality for many children. The anxiety that many children feel about their parents affects their ability to concentrate whilst in school. Some children leave early for this reason or phone parents during the day to check up on them. In the case of parental mental ill health, children have reported fearing that their parents will seriously harm themselves or attempt suicide whilst they are at school (Aldridge and Becker 2003).

For some children, school can be a great source of stability and distraction from their problems at home and many do very well at school (Frank 1995) and view it as a haven. Parents also appear to think school is important and children generally agree with this (Tunnard 2002a). However, some children do express a reluctance to confide in teachers and others who may be a potential source of support, as they fear poor responses from schools, including their privacy being compromised.

Emotional and behavioural development

Parents experiencing mood changes, withdrawing from those around them (including children), or the discord (or exaggerated intimacy) that can be associated with parental substance misuse or mental health problems can lead to children feeling fear, confusion or a sense of being in some way responsible. This can lead to behavioural difficulties or internalised emotional responses that are not readily observed or easily recognised.

If parental problems result in secrecy, for example about illegal drug use or criminal activities associated with it, where children hold information (which they often do even though sometimes their parents don't realise or acknowledge it) this can lead to children and young people feeling burdened and more separate from their friends and others from whom they must keep the secret.

Outcomes tend to be better when bad times are interspersed with good times in which children feel loved and well cared for. When negative experiences accumulate, or confused and inconsistent messages and care bring a sense of not being loved, impacts on children are worse (Kroll and Taylor 2003).

Hidden Harm (Gruer and Ainsworth 2003) cites the following potential impacts on children of problem drug use: emotional insecurity and impulsivity in young children; antisocial acts by boys; and depression, anxiety and withdrawal by girls. As children get older, conduct disorders, a risk of offending and alcohol or drug use become more likely; and in teenagers, a risk of self-blame, guilt and increased suicide risk have all been reported.

Parents with moderate mental health problems are more likely than non-affected parents to perceive behavioural problems in their child, with about a half to two-thirds of children's behaviour being seen by them as affected (Tunnard 2004). However, this is based on parental perceptions, which are likely to be influenced by parental confidence as well as competence.

Some of the behaviours that might manifest in children who are affected by parental mental health problems or substance misuse can be seen as coping mechanisms. The research into coping strategies for children in these circumstances is limited and relates to more generic adverse circumstances, such as parental disability and domestic violence. Gorin (2004) identifies four ways of coping that emerge from the literature and research available (see box below). These coping responses are more likely to emerge unconsciously than as deliberate strategies; and it is likely that ways of coping will change over time (Bancroft and others 2004).

Coping mechanisms of children and young people whose parents have mental health/substance misuse problems

Avoidance/distraction

This can include physically avoiding parents or the home environment, with many children finding a 'haven', such as a friend or family members' home or their own bedroom (Mullender and others 2002). Avoidance can also be psychological, with children ignoring or not thinking about their problems or pretending things are otherwise. Some children become loners or refuse to discuss their feelings. Others use distractions, such as music, TV, computers, or (more often for girls than boys) writing in diaries (Fuller and others 2000). Some children appear to throw themselves into their schoolwork or a hobby; and some deflect attention from their real lives by making things up to tell their peers about their home life (Barnard and Barlow 2003). Erickson and Henderson (1992) reported younger children talking to soft toys, pets and creating imaginary worlds.

Protection or inaction

Children can feel responsible for their parent's well-being or that of their siblings. One way this manifests itself in children is by them 'keeping watch' for signs of difficulty, which for some children can lead to staying away from school or avoiding going out. This is particularly noted in studies relating to parental mental health and to parental alcohol misuse. Girls are more commonly reported to take protective action in this way (Laybourn and others 1996). Where parental substance misuse is present, some children have spoken of hiding money or possessions and others of giving their parents money that they have saved for them. In all cases, when children don't take protective action they can experience feelings of guilt and distress about this, particularly (but not exclusively) when there is domestic violence or abuse of their siblings.

Confrontation/intervention/self-destruction

The most common way for children to intervene or confront their parents is by shouting at them (this is more likely than physical intervention in domestic violence situations). Some children dispense drugs, alcohol and/or medication to parents and others try psychological strategies to try and change their parent's behaviour or views, such as ridiculing them or appealing to them.

Help-seeking and action

Telling others about their situation or asking for advice from external sources is the second most common response by children (the most common being avoidance). Where children are able to discuss their situation this helps them to make sense of their own feelings and to be involved in considering the best way forward; both of which are factors known to increase their resilience. Unfortunately, when there is pressure to keep things secret within families, this undermines the potential for children to utilise this important coping behaviour.

Source: Gorin 2004

Identity

As children get older and become more curious about the world around them, developing clear likes, dislikes and opinions, there is a tendency for them to see themselves as being at the centre of everything. This is natural, but can be problematic when children have a disproportionate sense of their own impact and responsibility for what goes on around them. Where parental problems are seen as more clearly emanating from another source, for example when children view parental drinking as an 'illness', they are less likely to experience this sense of guilt and responsibility (Laybourn and others 1996). A fear of developing the same problems as their parents is common in children affected by either parental substance use or parental mental health problems. For example many professionals encounter children who have discussed their fear that mental illness is 'catching'.

Children and young people who have a clear sense of themselves as separate from their families and their problems tend to fare better than children who don't. Developing a view of themselves as valued and special is an important part of this and can potentially be undermined by inconsistent parenting where there is a lack of positive reinforcement. At worst this can lead to children lacking confidence and feeling 'unlovable' (Fahlberg 1991).

Identity problems can be compounded further for black and minority ethnic children and children of dual heritage. Depending on their family's attitude and behaviour, children could potentially have a clear sense of their gender, race and culture by the age of three or four (Bee

2000), but this will vary. However, children may sometimes internalise racist stereotypes from the wider society and misattribute their parent's substance-misuse to their ethnicity.

Family and social relationships

The impact on families of becoming isolated from extended families or wider networks of support has already been mentioned, but it is also possible for immediate family members to experience isolation from each other as a result of their difficulties. This can manifest itself in concrete ways, such as parental separation or divorce; or in more subtle ways, such as avoidance of each other or a lack of open communication.

There is often a tendency for parents to underplay their problems, either in an attempt to protect the child from knowing too much or as a result of denial. However, children often know more than their parents think they do and they pick up on things which, if denied, can lead to an increased sense of confusion and isolation. Such secrets and lies could be described as creating 'a world of mirrors where nothing is as it seems' (Kroll and Taylor 2003, p.184). If children (or partners) are not told the truth, and they suspect as much, they can experience this as rejection, become mistrustful and find their suspicions are raised further. Denial within families can cause a range of reactions in children such as anger, blame and conflict or alliances and splits within the family.

Difficulties in communication can also take the form of inappropriate comments being made to children by parents when they are distressed, angry or inebriated.

Changes in family members' roles in response to changing situations over time (such as one parent taking over the role of the 'unwell' parent or children taking on 'adult' tasks) can lead to children and young people struggling with new ways of relating to family members. Later, when a parent is more able to take the reins again, this may be resisted and lead to conflict.

Children's friendships outside the family can suffer due to stigma, not feeling they can bring friends home and the responsibilities of their caring role.

When faced with a crisis, some young people leave home prematurely; whereas others stay on longer than they might otherwise do, to support one or both parents or siblings. For young people who do wish to leave home, gaps in benefits can be prohibitive; similarly, for those who look after parents, a lack of financial resources and support can restrict access to some of the recreation and relaxation opportunities open to others.

Social presentation

The way in which children and young people present to others can be affected by parental difficulty. If there is poor hygiene or inappropriate dress due to neglect, children can appear different, experience bullying or show a lack of confidence. If parents model inappropriate behaviour or coping styles (such as aggression, substance use or criminal behaviour) and their children exhibit them, this will set them apart further resulting in people perceiving them negatively.

Self-care skills

Children and young people's self-care skills can similarly be reduced in these circumstances: a lack of guidance and support, or experiences of neglect, can result in a lack of self-esteem, low mood or lack of skills development. Conversely, the child undertaking caring responsibilities from a young age can heighten such skills.

Additional issues

Children as young carers

In a 1997 study, ChildLine found that where mothers had alcohol problems it was common for role reversal to occur whereby children took on a caring role. Dearden and Becker (2004) found that nearly a quarter of all children and young people who are considered to be young carers are looking after someone with mental health difficulties and are providing both practical and emotional care. They report that emotional care is the most demanding; and that they experience restrictions to their social life and stigma. Young carers may also have restricted life choices. It is important to acknowledge that there can be, and often are, positive aspects to being a young carer, with many feeling it to be a positive choice that bolsters their self-esteem, enhances their skills, maturity, relationships and emotional intelligence.

Whether or not they are undertaking practical or emotional care of their parents, many children often worry about parents to the exclusion of themselves. When asked how their parent's illness affected them, half the children in a recent study (reported by Tunnard 2004) referred only to concerns felt about their parent. Various studies have shown that children are more concerned about the issues relating to the emotional than the practical support of their parent.

Differing impact of various substances misused

Limited research has been done on the effects on parenting of the different types of drugs used. Famularo and others (1992) linked problem alcohol use with physical abuse by fathers and neglect by mothers. However, in her review of the literature and research, Tunnard (2002b) found that whilst the likelihood of children being at risk of neglect and emotional abuse tends to be increased, this is not generally the case for other forms of abuse. Forrester (2000) found in a localised study that over 60 per cent of children on the child protection register for neglect and emotional abuse had one or more substance-misusing parents.

Pre- and post-birth issues

During pregnancy, substance-misusing women are less likely to access services and are more likely to neglect their own health and diet, which in turn affects their own mental and physical preparation for the baby and the baby's health.

The effect on babies of different drugs used by their mothers in pregnancy is variable and multiple drug use complicates this further. In addition to the potential for low birth weights and premature births, complications can potentially be fundamental and long lasting. They can include: developmental delay, obstetric complications, muscular twitching, irritability, poor concentration, feeding difficulties, high-pitched crying, and reduced responsiveness.

The issue of detoxification in pregnancy is particularly complex. For example the use of methadone can potentially adversely impact on the baby's health, but the sudden cessation of drugs can also carry risks. Therefore medical supervision is very important in order for careful assessment and analysis of individual needs and circumstances to take place. There is a need for continued research to inform practice, but the weight of evidence and opinion suggests that, in pregnancy, maintaining methadone or 'stable' drug use may be preferable to detoxification.

Adult mental health problems can be exacerbated by, or even occur as a result of, pregnancy and childbirth; and in turn have an impact on the child. Postnatal depression and the more serious condition postpartum psychosis affect, respectively, 10–15 per cent of mothers and two in every thousand mothers. Evidence shows an association between postnatal depression and problematic mother–infant relationships, with potential for adverse cognitive and emotional impacts on the developing child. Post-partum psychosis can carry greater risks of suicidal or infanticidal thoughts, hallucinations and delusions (Falkov 1998), though this is rare.

Conclusion

The literature on the potential impact on children of parental mental health and substance misuse continues to grow and is useful in highlighting the sorts of issues faced by children and their families, and the practitioners and professionals working with them. Assessing the impact on individual children and families is a skilled and complex task, which relies on the analysis, reflection and self-awareness of those undertaking it to counter any assumptions or unchecked value judgements. A clear focus, which questions and explores the everyday experience of children and other family members (rather than an overemphasis on crisis or 'unusual' incidents), is needed; along with a child-focused ecological approach and knowledge of research and other evidence about effective or promising interventions. Approaches to assessment are considered further in Chapter 5.

3. What helps build resilience in these families?

Some children seem to be more affected by trauma in childhood than others. The term for the apparently increased ability to emerge from difficult situations without major negative impact on the individual is 'resilience'. This chapter considers factors that increase resilience and emphasises the importance of children being helped to sustain or develop a sense of self-efficacy and autonomy. It also considers familial and parenting characteristics that can enhance resilience.

This chapter goes on to consider cultural connectedness, values, and identity within the community, which can have positive effects on a child's resilience. It stresses that knowledge of resilience and all the points made above, when translated into practical support, can promote positive change.

The notion of 'resilience' within social care, particularly in relation to children's services, is a relatively new one but one that has gained increasing currency in the past decade. Services have for a long time tended to focus on vulnerable children in terms of the 'risks of significant harm' that they face or the 'needs' they have that are not being met at the time. This is still the case, although the emphasis, whether it be 'risk driven' or 'need driven', shifts over time. Currently there is a greater tendency (supported by the *Framework for Assessment of Children in Need and their Families*, Department of Health 2000; and more recently by the *Common Assessment Framework*, HM Government 2006b), to consider the strengths and protective factors within families. This raises the question of what strengths or factors within individuals, families or the wider life experience of children enable some to cope better with adverse experiences, unmet needs or risks than others? Also, why do some children who experience abuse or neglect, parental alcohol misuse, or who witness domestic violence appear to fare better than others who have had similar adverse experiences? What makes the difference? This apparently increased ability to emerge from difficult situations without major negative impacts on the individual is referred to as *resilience*.

Resilience factors operate at the level of the child, family and external environment. There are different manifestations of 'resilience', for example there are those who succeed despite high risk status; those who exhibit maturity and coping in the face of chronic stress; and those who have suffered extreme trauma but have recovered and prospered (Newman and Blackburn 2002). Resilience is not fixed but changes over time, often showing itself in later life following an earlier phase where difficulties in coping were exhibited. Whilst longitudinal studies show that many children recover from short-lived problems, when adversities are continuous and severe and there are no observable protective factors, resilience is much rarer.

> there is ... no simple association between stress and gain. Some stressors may trigger resilient assets in children, others may compound chronic difficulties. If children are subjected to a relentless stream of multiple adversities, negative consequences are highly likely to follow.
>
> (Newman and Blackburn 2002, p.4)

Poor early experiences don't necessarily dictate future outcomes, however, as compensatory interventions can trigger responses that enhance resilience.

For the purposes of this handbook and the Building Resilience project, the focus on resilience is synonymous with a focus on 'what's good for families' and especially 'what's good for the children within families'. It is concerned with what helps in minimising the impact of their difficulties and maximising the parent's opportunity to parent their child well enough and for the family to remain together. But this notion of resilience and a focus on it is not without its problems, and it is important to consider them here.

Firstly, if measures of 'resilience' focus on tangible but arbitrary aspects of an individual's apparent progress in life – such as doing well academically or securing employment, having a busy social life or sustaining a long-term relationship – then they may miss the less visible factors that may be at play. For instance, the apparently 'high achiever' may be viewed as having survived their early experiences relatively unscathed, when in fact their emotional life, confidence or self-esteem may be affected in ways that are neither seen, reported or considered. Equally, the lengths to which they have had to go in order to avoid some of the 'poorer outcomes' associated with adversity, may be great. It could be seen as minimising their struggle, or even offensive, to make statements that assume that in some way such individuals have been 'more resilient' or even 'coped better' than others.

Secondly, images that have been used to signify 'resilient children' as somehow 'unbreakable', 'bouncing back' or 'invulnerable' can be unhelpful (Rutter 1993, 1999) because resilience is relative, not absolute, and can change over time. Kroll and Taylor (2003) highlight the possibility of assumptions being made about a child that they are: 'once ok, always ok'. They discuss the potential for children who appear to be coping well at one time to be either concealing their difficulties or for their problems to be stored up for another time. At this point, they may become more vulnerable in a way that is compounded by their period of 'coping'. The positive labels of 'resilience' can therefore be as misleading as the negative ones.

Thirdly, in contrast to the above, those who experience mental health problems – such as depression or post-traumatic stress as a result of their experiences – can be seen as having an appropriate response to their situation. Their emotional reaction is perhaps, if viewed more positively, congruent, expressive and necessary. Such reactions may be a first step in helping some people to identify, question and move on from any damaging perceptions or self-beliefs that their experiences have left them with.

Fourthly, a focus on resilience could be interpreted as conferring too much responsibility on the person who has experienced the adversity, their 'hardiness' in relation to the adversity becoming the focus. This could in itself potentially compound any guilt, self-blame and sense of over responsibility that individuals may experience.

Finally, Newman and Blackburn (2002) raise the issue of the tension that can occur between 'protection' and 'resilience' – to some extent, resilience can often be seen as occurring as a result of exposure to stress. They therefore suggest that an over-concentration on identifying and eliminating risk factors could potentially weaken children's capacity to overcome adversity. They would argue that gradual exposure to life's stresses at a manageable level (this would be hard to gauge) could help people/children develop a resistance to adverse reactions to stress. Nonetheless, experiences that could be seen to promote resilience would not always be socially acceptable. In relation to child protection issues, if children were left to cope with some situations in order to 'build their resistance to adversity', this would be extremely contentious, potentially very dangerous and clearly unethical. But it is important to acknowledge that all interventions, even when (or perhaps especially when) their purpose is to protect, can either harm or help. A useful perspective to help with such dilemmas can be to remind ourselves that the purpose of services and interventions should be to elicit the internal strengths, resilience, motivations and goals that already exist within individuals and families.

Also, given some of the other concerns about the notion of resilience, it is important to be clear in our thinking and in what we communicate when we talk about resilience with other professionals, in reports and with families. It is not so much about someone's capacity to manage, as about the associations between the presence of some factors (often referred to as 'protective factors') with long-term good outcomes.

To assess resilience factors alongside risks, and to give full consideration to factors and inverventions likely to promote resilience and reduce risks, increases the opportunity for establishing a way forward that is, comprehensive, evidence-informed and promotes 'best possible' outcomes. Such a focus can help reduce the sorts of 'additional harm' that can compound difficult experiences, perhaps needlessly, when some attention given to an aspect of someone's life or needs could relieve their situation or distress. The risk/ vulnerability matrix on page 55 provides a useful framework for this.

Much work has been done to explore what factors seem to support the resilience of individuals and these factors will be described in the following sections. However, it is not enough to identify what factors are associated with resilience. This information only becomes useful if such factors can be affected, and such knowledge can be translated into effective service responses, support or interventions for children and families.

Factors that increase resilience

The parenting, familial and community factors that seem to improve outcomes, if present for children and young people, are considered separately in this section. In reality these factors often overlap.

Much of the literature and research about resilience or 'protective factors' (a term often used interchangeably with 'resilience factors') has focused on adversity in a general sense, though it is still relevant for children affected specifically by parental mental health or parental substance misuse. Newman and Blackburn (2002), in their international study, found that common factors could be seen across cultural and geographical boundaries. Other research has been more specific, such as Velleman's (1993 and 2004) work on outcomes for children of alcohol-misusing parents. A range of sources has been drawn on to compile the lists of resilience-enhancing factors below, including Velleman and Orford (1993 and 1999), Newman and Blackburn (2002), Tunnard (2002a), Bancroft and others (2004), Kroll and Taylor (2003) and Cleaver and others (1999).

Factors that enhance children's resilience

Positive relationship with a family member or parental figure

For all children and young people facing difficulties of any kind, supportive family members are the most powerful positive factor influencing their ability to cope. This is due both to the attachment relationship, which provides the child with the foundation for their self-esteem and for developing relationships with others, and to the increased likelihood of them receiving the care and support they need practically and emotionally.

The presence of at least one unconditionally supportive parent or parent substitute is key. This enables children and young people to develop what Fonagy and others (1994) refer to as a 'reflective self-function' (which they define as having an awareness of mental processes in oneself and in others, and the ability to take account of one's own mental states and those of others to understand why people behave in certain ways – in other words thinking about yourself in relation to others). Whilst the parent or parents who are experiencing substance misuse or mental health problems may provide the child with much of this understanding, the research indicates that the presence of another adult improves outcomes. Such adults do not necessarily have to live with the child, but need to be an integral and influential part of their lives. Often the partner of the parent who has the most difficulties is concerned about, or supporting, their partner. Their attention can be drawn away from the child, so this lends weight to the crucial need to support the 'least vulnerable' parent to bolster their ability to provide essential attention to the child.

Influence of another stable adult figure or figures

Beyond the child's family or home environment, the presence of a committed mentor or positive and interested adult outside the family is also an important positive factor. Such a relationship can provide the child or young person with encouragement: much needed attention, consistency, a sense of stability and more. This may come from either informal networks such as members of the wider family, neighbours or friends' parents or from more formal sources such as teachers or other professionals. Such people can be an important source of support to parents by either giving them a break through the relief of knowing someone else is helping the child, or by providing a stabilising influence on the parent.

Positive social support networks and a social role

Support networks such as friendships, clubs, and membership of groups or attendance at faith-based institutions can all help children develop a sense of being valued or 'valuable'. Participation in extracurricular activities, which children enjoy or are good at, can promote their self-esteem. Similarly, the opportunity for older children (through voluntary or part-time work or membership of supportive groups or organisations) to 'make a difference' by helping others, enhances their self-esteem, social skills and the development of a positive identity.

Positive experiences away from the home can counter some of the stress or difficulty that some children face, giving them 'compensatory' moments of pleasure, fun and relaxation and something to look forward to. Having the opportunity to find out about how other people respond to them and to explore interests and skills in such settings, are all important in forming a sense of identity.

Positive school experiences

This is linked with the above two points in terms of the opportunity schools provide for forming friendships with peers, with other adults and for developing social skills, interests, talents and self-esteem. Educational success is an additional factor, which if experienced is associated with children who fare better later in life due to the opportunities it gives them, as well as to the increased self-esteem, knowledge and ways of understanding the world that help them to interact more positively within it.

A sense that one's own efforts can make a difference

For children as well as adults, their problems are likely to have a more negative impact on them if they feel helpless and that nothing is within their control. If they can be enabled to exert any influence on their own circumstances, however small, this can enhance their well-being. Being helped to make choices, and being consulted and asked about what they think will help them or what is important to them, can all promote their sense that they can make a difference. This links in with another important factor: the capacity to recognise and acknowledge the beneficial effects of adversity (as well as the damaging aspects). This may seem strange, but most people can relate to a sense that people often have when they have been through difficult times, that something within them has 'grown' or developed as a result. Whilst negative experiences aren't to be minimised, the impact of all experiences is mixed; and to acknowledge the positive can be affirming and help growth. Also, a sense that problems can be overcome is very important to young people becoming proactive and optimistic in their approach to life.

Personal or 'inherent' qualities

Children with good verbal skills, good cognitive ability, the absence of neurobiological problems, and who demonstrate autonomy, sociability and good self-esteem, tend to fare better than children who do not have these qualities. The extent to which some of these 'qualities' can be influenced varies of course, and the absence of some of the factors may be compounded or caused by the problems children have faced in their lives. A child's behaviour, confidence and ability is not static, however. With support and opportunities, some children who are regarded as 'unsociable' or 'inarticulate' for example, may demonstrate significant changes over time.

A child's own 'coping' skills

The more children are able to understand and express their feelings, the more they can make sense of their situations and survive them with less harm done. In families where feelings are denied, where emotions are seen as volatile or silenced, it is much harder for children to develop such positive responses. Interventions that bolster a child's ability to recognise and name feelings, as well as to express them and ask for help, will enhance their resilience. Some social situations and opportunities, such as activities that are challenging but achievable, can also provide children with opportunities to develop coping skills.

A child's view of themselves

Children who see themselves as separate from the problems in their family tend to fare better than those who believe that they are a part of the problems and that their problems are a part of them. Children whose parents are distressed, unwell or intoxicated or in withdrawal, often, and understandably, think that they are somehow compounding or causing the problems that they see around them. Some children at times blame themselves for their parents' state, or internalise their parents' feelings as being somehow about something they are or are not doing. Also, children feel the stigma that such families experience. They can feel alienated and judged and go on to internalise these negative views. Children who, while knowing they are part of a family, see themselves as distinct individuals with separate feelings, qualities and potential, are likely to have better outcomes.

Plans for the future

Children who can imagine their futures and who are encouraged and supported to make positive plans about their future are more likely to do well. Plans in the short term are also important as they provide things to look forward to, both with and without the rest of their family.

31

Early and compensatory experiences

Where a parent has discrete episodes of mental illness with fairly high functioning in between episodes, this appears to increase the opportunity for resilience in the child, whereas those whose parents' problems are chronic and enduring are more negatively affected. Also, the older the child is at the onset of their parent's mental health problems, the greater the range of coping resources they will have developed by the time the problems start. Therefore less early exposure to problems increases their life chances.

Similarly for children of substance-misusing parents, the absence of early loss and trauma will have given them the opportunity to develop their coping resources. Where there are substantial periods in which parents care for them well and they feel loved, they will fare better than if neglect is chronic and long term. Conversely, where levels of care and support differ significantly over time, with such changes making no sense to the child and messages about the value of the child being confusing, this will be more detrimental to children.

Familial and parenting characteristics that enhance resilience

A confiding relationship with a partner or with others

When parents under stress have a partner who they can share their thoughts, feelings and experiences with and with whom they can be honest, their well-being and in turn their parenting capacity is enhanced. For lone parents or parents in less positive relationships, it is important to find a confidante elsewhere. Also, parents who have positive relationships with others are more likely to be able to develop a positive attachment with their child. Being able to listen to their partners or others and reciprocate within relationships enhances this further.

Cohesive parental relationship

The absence of parental conflict is associated with better outcomes for children. If parents are able to present a 'united front' to their children, showing that they agree and are consistent in the boundaries they set and the plans they have, this helps children by providing the consistency they need and reducing confusion, insecurity and uncertainty. Consistently enforced rules are another resilience factor within parenting; and a cohesive relationship (where there is more than one parent) will support this.

Parental self-esteem

Parents who (with or without support) are able to value themselves and see what their positive qualities and abilities are and what they mean to other people are better able to parent effectively. Therefore interventions and informal support that seek to enhance (rather than undermine) self-esteem are very important.

Social life, rituals and routines

Parents who have regular contact with other adults or families who they value and who they enjoy being with is associated with greater resilience. Such opportunities, all too often lacking for families under stress, can enhance self-esteem and reduce stress. Obviously if socialising tends to reinforce problematic drinking or substance use, or is with people or in settings that increase anxiety, this becomes detrimental, but enhancing the positive social opportunities available is important.

If families can manage to do some things together – such as going to the park or sitting down for a family meal together – these positive and reliable experiences can enhance relationships, children's self-esteem and outlook, and give positive memories. Observing special occasions and rituals that were previously adhered to, such as all gathering together while a child opens their birthday presents, is important even when (and especially because) life is chaotic and littered with crises.

Adequate finances and employment opportunities

Families who have sufficient finances available to them fare better than those who don't. Increased resources mean more access to support for individuals within the family or for the whole family. These resources include more suitable housing; social and leisure opportunities; breaks and respite; private counselling; and access to support with childcare or even with domestic tasks. Where there is parental substance misuse, some of the areas of potential concern, such as finances being directed into drugs rather than in meeting children's basic needs, are mitigated if resources are more plentiful. However, this may mean in some families that it is easier to hide substance use, meaning some of the more emotional impacts on children, for example secrecy and denial, are harder to pick up.

Employment can obviously be one way of enhancing the finances of some families and part-time work for women with mental health problems is known to be a protective factor but, conversely, full-time work for women with young children increases the risks of parental stress impacting negatively on children.

Constructive coping styles and deliberate parental actions to minimise adversity for children

The coping strategies employed by parents impact directly or indirectly on the way the child manages their experiences and emotions. Tunnard (2002a) reported on a Scottish study, which demonstrated this link in families where parents were depressed. For example, if the parent had a non-productive coping style or avoided their problems (worrying, not talking about problems, self-blaming or wishful thinking) and was therefore less likely to seek help, their children tended to do the same. Conversely, if parents were more productive (focusing on positives, dealing with problems, seeking help), children did the same.

Some parents are proactive in trying to minimise the impact of their problems on their children. Parents who have experienced mental health problems over time and have come to know what helps and hinders their well-being often develop strategies to minimise the stress on them and to get support when they need it. Tunnard (2002a) reported on some of the strategies adopted by substance-misusing parents, which included planned separations as a way of protecting the child from their drug use or inability to care sufficiently well for them at the time. Often this meant the child spending time with relatives (frequently maternal grandmothers) for a period instead. Other strategies included safe storage of equipment; keeping other drug users out of the home; or having rules about not using drugs when the children were around. These strategies worked better for some people than others. Other strategies adopted by parents to reduce their own health problems arising from their drug use and, in turn, reduce the negative impact on their parenting included not taking drugs daily, getting enough sleep, eating properly, taking iron tablets and trying to avoid stress.

Parental substance misuse in itself can be viewed as a coping strategy when it has developed as a way of numbing feelings or avoiding problems. It is important that if people are being encouraged to reduce or abstain from substance or alcohol use that alternative coping strategies are explored.

Receiving treatment

There is some evidence that going into treatment for substance problems and using a substitute such as methadone can be a significant protective factor, leading to far greater stability, predictability of daily life and reduction of the distractions, secrecy and denial that impact on parenting and on children. Some parents, however, fear that if they use substitutes they will develop another addiction (Tunnard 2002a).

Receiving treatment or therapy for any psychological difficulty can mean raising memories and feelings that have been buried or denied as a coping mechanism, so undergoing treatment for complex problems linked with substance misuse or mental health problems can have an impact that is potentially negative in the shorter term. Ultimately, however, if such interventions are made in timely fashion, and if they are followed through by the individual concerned, they should promote resilience.

Openness and good communication

Whatever the nature of the problems within families, if there is an atmosphere of openness in which thoughts, feelings and uncertainties can be safely expressed, the outcomes for children (and the wider family) will be supported by this.

A knowledge of 'protective factors'

It is logical and has been demonstrated (Velleman 2004) that if parents know about the things that make a difference to children and to the outcomes for them, they are more able to utilise them. Helping parents to recognise the importance of certain factors, such as children's engagement in hobbies or the importance of observing family occasions and keeping some routines, is helpful and potentially empowering.

Community factors that enhance resilience

Cultural connectedness, values and identity

Families who see themselves as part of their community, who are linked in with groups and services, fare better than those who are disconnected, as already discussed in Chapter 2. For example if a positive identity or valued local culture exists within a community, or a family identifies positively as members of an ethnic or religious group, this relates to better outcomes and a more positive individual and family identity.

A socially rich environment in which people are inclined to look out for each other, intervene and help out is associated with better outcomes for children and families, as are good community resources such as accessible childcare, healthcare, transport, leisure and education facilities.

Bolstering resilience

As stated earlier, knowledge of resilience or 'protective' factors is not in itself enough to influence the experiences of children. However, if such knowledge is translated into support and actions aimed directly at influencing such factors, this can promote positive change. At the individual level, this could mean placing more emphasis on facilitating a child's access to a supportive adult, social or leisure opportunity or helping a parent understand and act on the knowledge of what is important for their child. When it comes to planning and shaping services, such knowledge adds weight to the importance of supporting extended family members, working more proactively with fathers and linking responses more effectively with schools or community resources. As, on the whole, the literature shows informal support to be more helpful to families than formal professional involvement, it is also worth services considering how they can better:

> *foster the characteristics of responsiveness, flexibility, reliability and supportiveness that characterise family and community supports*

> (Olsen and Wates 2003, p.26)

Some resilience factors are more amenable to influence than others and it would be naïve to suggest that a focus on boosting resilience factors alone will fully address the problems that many families face. However, an awareness of resilience factors and a weighing up of these alongside a consideration of needs, risks and potential for change will enhance assessments and could give rise to more appropriate interventions.

4. Professional responses and barriers to effective practice

This chapter explores the barriers, at the practice and strategic levels, to effective responses by services.

It considers the practice level, where too few professionals think about the family, the impacts of one member on another, and opportunities to promote and use the support of friends and family members. It looks at the lack of interagency knowledge-sharing; and the uncertainty amongst professionals as to how and where to access specific knowledge and expertise. It suggests that a greater focus on critical reflection and support with analysis is needed. It goes on to consider why some service responses are proving unhelpful, including the lack of focus on fathers, and some of the reasons why families may be reluctant to use a service.

This chapter also considers the strategic level, and why services are often organised around discrete areas – such as 'mental health' or 'substance misuse' – despite these not being separate and distinct for individuals and families. It suggests that more integrated working needs to be instigated, while keeping to tight budgets and appropriate levels of access to services.

Barriers to effective practice: What gets in the way?

This chapter explores, in more depth, some of the key practice issues of relevance to those providing support and services on an individual or family level.

Chapter 1 discussed the general tendency towards too little or late intervention sometimes leading to more extreme responses further down the line. Whilst some of these issues, such as the lack of talking therapies available for those with mild or moderate mental health difficulties, can be seen as linked to a lack of resources, others are directly affected by deficits in practitioner awareness, knowledge, training and confidence. These issues are discussed in Part 1 of this chapter.

Chapter 1 also established that the way in which services currently respond to families affected by parental mental health problems and substance misuse is variable and that there is a lack of preventative and early intervention services (despite policy drivers aimed at promoting them). There are also significant barriers to providing coordinated support across relevant professional disciplines, with interagency working difficulties being rife and perhaps the hardest factor to overcome. Part 2 of this chapter focuses entirely on such issues, which are most appropriately and meaningfully addressed at a strategic level.

Raising awareness and challenging stigma

The nature and impact of stigma

having a mental illness is one of the most overtly stigmatised attributes an individual can have, rivalled only by substance abuse or homelessness

(Link, Phelan and others 1999 in Hinshaw 2005, p.716)

The stigmatisation of people with mental health problems and substance misuse issues is well documented, and its significance and impact on families has been discussed to some extent earlier in this book. Stigmatisation does not occur as a result of the presence of mental illness or substance misuse, but as a result of the discriminatory attitudes and responses of wider society to them.

Experiences of stigmatisation compound people's difficulties significantly and can limit opportunities, such as their access to housing, employment, medical care and insurance coverage (Corrigan 2004), and is the greatest barrier to social inclusion for people with mental health problems (Social Exclusion Unit 2004). Stigma can also limit the availability of research funding, access to treatment, and attainment of personal relationships and educational and vocational goals (Sartorius 1998).

Both substance misuse and mental health problems are not necessarily visible, so stigma and (perceived or anticipated) negative attitudes can lead people to conceal their diagnosis or difficulties and make them less likely to ask for help or admit to the nature of their problems. The negative media portrayal of those who misuse substances and those with mental health problems as dangerous or potentially violent (Wahl 1995) further influences public perception and, in turn, the view that those with mental health or substance use problems have about others and about themselves. As Hinshaw puts it, prejudice, stereotyping and discrimination are related, but stigma:

incorporates all these processes but transcends them by including the strong likelihood that the castigated individual will internalise the degradation

(Hinshaw 2005, p.715)

Unfortunately, most of the relevant literature and research relating to people with mental health or substance misuse issues focuses on the negative rather than any positive aspects of people or their lives.

whilst nearly all of the relevant literature has emphasised family burden – relating to the negative effects of coping with a relative with mental illness – anecdotal evidence suggests that in at least in a subset of families, the experience has fostered sensitivity, courage, and a more positive outlook on life

(Hinshaw 2005, p.721)

Part 1: The practice level

Awareness/knowledge and confidence

The reasons for a lack of awareness (of issues that if better understood would enhance practice responses) are complex, but in part, the separation of services means too few relevant practitioners and professionals think in terms of family relationships and the impacts of one member on another. The pattern of client contact within adult drug services and in some adult mental health settings, for example, makes it easy to lose sight of the needs (or even the presence or relevance) of the adult's child or children. Some agencies discourage adult users from bringing children into the office (or service setting) because facilities aren't 'suitable' or because of understandable concerns that the child's presence will impinge on what can be discussed. However in making such decisions or responses, agencies should consider far more than simple issues of 'practicality', since this approach may critically skew what is looked at (in terms of needs of the family) and significantly narrow the focus of what is seen or noticed by the professional.

Kroll and Taylor (2003) interviewed practitioners from a range of the relevant settings and found that many of those working with adults felt that parenting capacity was not something they could assess. Furthermore, there was often ambivalence or uncertainty among them (and it seems likely to be the case for many non-statutory children's services as well) about making referrals to statutory children and families social work teams for them to assess parenting capacity and needs. Many were unsure about when or how to make a referral and, in particular, whether or not they were able to make an informal enquiry without 'triggering the might of the child protection machinery' (p.225).

Conversely, many children's services practitioners consider parental mental health problems or substance misuse to be specialist areas falling outside their expertise. Neither do they appear, however, to be involving (or to be successful in attempts to involve) relevant adult workers within their processes as often as they could. Forrester and Harwin (2006) found substance use workers to be conspicuously absent from interagency meetings, for example.

The extent to which working in this way, solely with individuals, has become fixed in many services should not be underestimated. For many practitioners and professionals used to working in centres with adults only, visiting people at home or working across family boundaries can be perceived, for example, as unethical or potentially damaging to professional/ adult service user relationships or confidentiality.

That said, increased knowledge and confidence can only be advantageous for practice. Whilst no one professional discipline can hold expertise or knowledge in all relevant issues, better awareness of where and with whom expertise or knowledge is held and how to access it is essential.

So it seems that, before the knowledge gaps of relevant professionals can be addressed, there is a need for increased awareness and appreciation of the systemic nature of family functioning – the impact that one family member and their needs and behaviour has on another – as well as a clearer message within organisations that *supporting families* is everybody's responsibility.

Mental health awareness

Tunnard (2004) highlighted the need for a greater understanding of mental health issues and for all professionals to understand that the vast majority of people with mental health problems don't harm or neglect their children; and that fluctuations in their parenting capacity could in many cases be accommodated by flexible services. Also, practitioners and professionals need to value and recognise the importance of wider family and friends more; and to utilise and promote such sources of support more routinely in their work with families.

Drug and alcohol awareness

Velleman (2004), in his work concerning substance misuse, discussed the need for those working with children in all settings to be made aware of the possible signs and symptoms that can manifest themselves in children who are adversely affected by parental substance use or other parental problems – such as behaviour and emotional difficulties, school problems, difficulty with transitions to adolescence, and 'precocious maturity'. He also argued the need for a greater awareness of resilience factors among professionals and parents.

The nature of substance misuse and responses to it are developing all the time, so there is a particular challenge in raising the awareness and confidence of relevant professionals in this area. Forrester and Harwin (2006) identified a need for more training around substance misuse for social workers in child care. Lack of confidence was raised, by Kroll and Taylor (2003), as potentially contributing to the reasons for a lack of joint intervention, along with professional 'fears of exposing one's practice' to professionals from other disciplines.

In their work with two local authorities, Hart and Powell (2006) also identified that both social workers and referrers appeared to lack an understanding of the complexity of assessing the impact of, and the needs arising from, parental drug misuse. A number of referrals, case notes and reports said no more than 'drug use by parents'; and gave no adequate consideration or information to critically consider the variables of the individual family situation. This was often done without consulting drug workers who may have had expertise to offer. They also found that many workers had naïve views about drugs and tended to overemphasise abstinence as being required rather than having a clear and critical focus on children's needs. Elliot and Watson (1998) highlighted that many parents think workers don't know enough about their difficulties or about polydrug use, and focus too narrowly on heroin use.

Assessment issues

There is often a lack of clear analytical assessment of families' needs, with a tendency for repeated initial assessments to take place following single incidents of concern (Hart and Powell 2006); and often no core assessments until increased professional intervention is necessitated through the family situation worsening. When assessments do take place they tend to be undertaken on a single agency basis with inadequate consultation with other relevant professionals. Plans for interventions often fail to utilise the network of potential support and input. Hart and Powell (2006) found partnership working to be underdeveloped, with little use being made of network meetings or family group conferences.

Social work assessments that take place within the *Framework for Assessment of Children in Need and their Families* (Department of Health 2000) have often been found to lack narrative; to be parent-focused, with children being less visible than they ought to be; and to lack transparent and clear analysis (Dalzell and Sawyer 2007, Hart and Powell 2006). This is not just true of assessments relating to families affected by parental mental health issues or substance misuse but of all family assessments: the struggle to establish what is 'good enough' in terms of parenting, when significant harm is indicated, and how to achieve good outcomes within resource constraints applies to them all. Yet poor assessments take almost as much, if not the same amount of time and energy as good ones. A greater focus on critical reflection and support with analysis is needed and, ultimately, may well reduce the efforts required by professionals.

Decision-making

Decision-making often happens almost by default. Kroll and Taylor (2003) found that factors that influenced assessments and decisions – not necessarily consciously at the time – include the reputation of the family, a fear of making judgements when there is poverty, and anxiety about the impact of child protection work. They also found a tendency for professionals to feel relieved when some families withdrew from services, and to be more disposed to close such cases or withdraw the service in response to apparent withdrawal. The lack of clear analysis and critical consideration of family circumstances over time can, and often does, lead to decisions and interventions that occur almost 'by accident'. Such cases include children becoming 'looked after' in crisis, but at a time when the situation is no longer amenable to change – so they end up remaining away from home after months of uncertainty. When kinship carers look after the child, this lack of clear planning, direction and support can place greater strain on the placement too. Hollows (2003) used the term 'creeping judgements' to describe these kinds of situation – where, for example, a series of short-term, 'duty' responses set the pattern and nature of long-term intervention, even though they are often based on single incidents or 'snapshot' assessments.

Unhelpful service responses

Assessing what support is needed by families, and finding the resources or skills to provide whatever is necessary, are not easy tasks. However, some approaches seem particularly unhelpful, such as the use of 'warning letters' in which it is 'threatened' that assessments will take place if further incidents are heard of or referrals received, or offering early morning appointments and then closing the case if a family doesn't attend. Such practices are seen as an intervention and yet they don't facilitate an assessment taking place and potentially hinder current or future engagement with some families. It is not surprising that many professionals, not used to taking a whole-family approach, perhaps do not know how to intervene for the best and are more likely to rely on more mechanised uncritical responses, which seem 'safer', regardless of their effectiveness. Jack (1997) suggests that a 'risk and blame culture' had led to 'less support for social workers to take risks in developing more supportive approaches in working with families'.

Much is often made by professionals of parents 'refusing services' or 'failing to admit their problems'. Hamer (2005) argues that such statements are labelling and are often based on professionals' notions of 'support', when what families are actually refusing are interventions that don't meet their needs. These may, in the view of parents, have intended or unintended consequences, which place greater strain on their families or which they don't understand because they have not been generated through any meaningful collaboration with them. Services are often offered by professionals suggesting to parents that they are not managing or that things need to change or improve. This can make it very hard for some parents to accept what is being offered as it may be construed as an admission of 'not coping', which brings a whole range of anxieties, many valid, with it.

Parental 'resistance' to intervention and support is not necessarily caused by professional ways of working and is common among people experiencing addictions. However, apart from substance misuse workers, most professionals get little or no preparation within their training for working with denial, minimisation, avoidance or aggression and this makes them less likely to respond in ways that reduce resistance. In fact much of the way in which child protection work is conducted would seem likely to increase resistance.

Lack of focus on fathers

A tendency within social care and family support services to focus interventions on mothers and to exclude fathers can reduce the usefulness of practice and services. In assessments of need as well as within interventions, the focus, even when initially targeted at the whole family, quickly shifts to a focus on the mother (Ryan 2000). This means that not only do fathers miss out on the opportunity to better understand and meet their children's needs, but that mothers are ascribed the lion's share of responsibility for changing family circumstances. Another potential impact of this is to fail to provide support for (or even to collude with) situations where mothers or children are afraid of fathers, for example where there is domestic violence. As Kroll and Taylor (2003) point out, if professionals are reticent about approaching fathers, this must disempower mothers further. This failure to include fathers as a matter of course, further undermines a whole-family approach that could improve the effectiveness of interventions.

Practical arrangements

The practical arrangements within which many services operate can also be seen as hindering effective practice, for example a lack of flexibility about where and when appointments can take place. This can mean that some parents who are already known to be struggling with structure or appointments are potentially being 'set up to fail' if only offered early morning appointments or if they are given lots of appointments at different places (and especially if these are without adequate facilities for their children). In some cases, this is perhaps deliberate – some 'testing out' often occurs within the social work relationship and can provide useful information – but with some parents it could also reduce the possibility of securing a trusting constructive relationship and of moving forward. Waiting times for appointments and assessments, a lack of mutual trust and a fear of children being removed are all further barriers to the take-up of services by parents.

Part 2: The strategic level

Complex range of 'single-user' services

Where there are parental mental health problems, the affected parent might be eligible for an assessment and services from an adult mental health team. Their child, if they have their own needs or difficulties, may have their needs assessed by a children and families social work team or a Child and Adolescent Mental Health Service (CAMHS). Similarly, there are separate teams and services set up to assess and provide services for adults with substance misuse issues. Sometimes these are also aimed at those with problem alcohol use and at other times these are separate. Add in providers of education, community care services, health, therapeutic support, housing, probation and Connexions or other targeted youth support services and any one family could have a large number of agencies involved at one time. There are exceptions, as some services are set up with the whole family in mind, but these tend more often than not to be voluntary sector services and even these services are usually one of a number of agencies involved in a family's life. Conversely, with no single route for support and differing realms of 'responsibility' within services, some individuals and families do not receive the support they require, with different services each thinking they are the responsibility of another.

Whilst services are often organised around discrete areas of need such as 'mental health' or 'substance use', the needs of individuals and families are not separate and distinct. They often come with multiple problems such as poverty, child behavioural issues, dual diagnosis or domestic violence, and one area of difficulty compounds another, making such distinctions potentially misleading.

Lack of effective joint working

Parental substance misuse and mental ill health jointly highlight and are affected by the gaps between adults and children's services and more generally in interagency working, with services often failing to coordinate an effective response to multiple issues within one family. It is therefore perhaps not surprising that at the first workshop in the Building Resilience project participants overwhelmingly gave the same response to the question: *What would you like to see change or improve in relation to services for people affected by parental mental health issues or substance misuse?* Their response: more integrated working.

There are a number of reasons for the lack of an effective joined-up response to family needs by services. The Social Care Institute for Excellence (SCIE) in their report *Alcohol, Drug and Mental Health Problems: Working with families* (Kearney and others 2003) identified the following causes/reasons for a lack of integrated responses.

- Discussion and clarification between agencies with different remits about their methods, terms of reference, values and priorities, are needed if agencies are to fully understand one another and complement what each other do. However, this level of ongoing communication and relationship-building is time consuming and this can be prohibitive. Also such differences can lead to misunderstandings and tensions, and sometimes to a resulting lack of motivation to work more closely together.
- When policies and procedures only focus on single users and fail to cater for multiple areas of need within the same individual or family this can hinder, or at least fail to support, an integrated response.

Financial constraints and high eligibility thresholds

All agencies are operating within budgetary constraints and the need to stretch limited resources leads to increasingly tighter 'gatekeeping' measures, such as eligibility thresholds that limit those who can access a particular service to those with the perceived highest need. In the mental health field, for example, this often means that mental health difficulties need to be regarded as 'severe and enduring' before a service user can access a service. In children and families statutory social work teams, the level of need encountered by a child often has to be quite high in many teams, verging on them being 'in need of protection', before assessments are undertaken.

Another reason the SCIE review identified a lack of effective joint working is that commissioning arrangements for smaller non-statutory agencies tend to be short term, with budgets only provided for a year or two at a time. Much time and energy is spent within such agencies trying to demonstrate the effectiveness of what they do in order to help secure the next round of funding. The consequence is that joint working arrangements are not as well developed as they could be.

Lack of data collection

The data collection systems currently being operated do not measure and capture the size of the problem effectively, if at all. Until local statutory and voluntary agencies routinely and consistently have a record of how many parents and children are affected by parental mental health or substance misuse issues and what their presenting needs are, the significance of these issues to services and the prioritisation of resources into these areas is unlikely to occur.

Black and minority ethnic groups: A lack of accessible services

There is strong evidence that black and minority ethnic (BME) groups receive fewer services or services which are of poorer quality and effectiveness than white service users. Research from the PricewaterhouseCoopers group, undertaken for the DfES (2006b), suggests that most local authorities are struggling to engage with BME groups effectively. They found BME parents showed increased reluctance to seek information and support through state services, had a greater fear of stigmatisation and were less likely to feel engaged with mainstream schools and services aimed at supporting parents.

Kurtz and others (2005), in their research for Young Minds into the needs and experiences of services for BME young people with mental health problems, found that it was very rare to find specialist Child and Adolescent Mental Health Services that were comprehensively responding to the needs of local communities. Young people from minority ethnic groups were not likely to access services until a late stage when they were in crisis. They also commented that staff groups are rarely representative of the ethnic diversity of the communities they are based within and, when there were black and minority ethnic staff, they are often informally placed in a role of being the 'BME specialist' and are poorly supported in this. They conclude that all efforts towards 'good practice' are only effective in as far as services are taken up. If services are not accessible and acceptable to all, they are failing in a significant part of their core purpose.

All the above findings are confirmed by SCIE's research briefing *Black and Minority Ethnic Parents with Mental Health Problems and their Children* (Greene and others 2008), which found that mental health problems among these groups, compounded by lack of adequate treatment responses and support, can have enduring adverse effects upon their children.

Mental health

In relation specifically to mental health, there is a large body of evidence of failures to provide equal access and opportunity to black and minority ethnic service users. *Delivering Race Equality: A framework for action – Mental health services* (Department of Health 2003b) showed the following experiences of inequality to be in evidence:

- problems in accessing services
- lower satisfaction with services generally and with hospital care
- cultural and language barriers
- lower levels of general practitioner involvement in people's overall care
- inadequate community-based crisis care
- lower incidence of user involvement
- inadequate support for black community initiatives
- higher compulsory admission rates
- higher involvement in legal and forensic systems of intervention
- higher transfer rates to medium and high security facilities
- higher voluntary admission rates to hospital
- reduced effectiveness of hospital treatment and longer hospital stays
- less likelihood of having broad needs addressed within treatment/care planning process
- more severe and coercive treatments
- lower access to talking treatments.

Similarly the national census (conducted by the Healthcare Commission in 2005), which obtained feedback from 34,000 people who were using mental health services, found Black African and Caribbean people to be three times more likely to be admitted to hospital and up to 44 per cent more likely to be detained under the Mental Health Act, with Black Caribbean men more likely to be restrained than any other group. A *British Journal of Psychiatry* study (Leese and others 2006) also found that black patients were over-represented (by eight times) in high security psychiatric hospitals; and were likely to be younger on admission and to have had more previous hospital admissions, suggesting a pattern of 'revolving door contact' (Lyall 2006). Research by the Sainsbury Centre for Mental Health into 'the costs of race inequality' indicated that the over-representation of these groups in psychiatric hospitals, secure services and some community services costs up to a £100m a year in London; money which could more appropriately be invested in community-based services (Sainsbury Centre for Mental Health 2006).

Substance misuse

In relation to adults with substance misuse issues, there are some differences between different ethnic groups in both their patterns of drug use and the services they access. Abdulrahim (2006) reports that the overall prevalence of drug use among BME populations is lower than among the white population in the UK. Usage appears to be particularly low among South Asians and Black Africans. Black Caribbean drug use is thought to be on a par with white drug use, with the prevalence of cannabis use bringing the numbers up. African and Caribbean users are more likely to present to services with crack cocaine problems and with problematic cannabis use, whereas heroin is more likely to be used among South Asian people who have problematic drug use. Low needle exchange uptake is therefore of concern. Little is known about newly arriving communities, although some knowledge is emerging about the use of khat (or qat) among Somali communities.

With these differences taken into account, Abdulrahim reports that all BME groups are under-represented within treatment services throughout the country.

Abdulrahim summarises the barriers to uptake of drug treatment by BME groups as being:

- a denial of drug use in some communities (by communities and professionals alike)
- a fear of confidentiality being breached
- the unrepresentative ethnicity of staff
- a lack of understanding by staff of cultural factors
- a lack of an appropriate service response
- an underdeveloped treatment for crack addiction
- a lack of cannabis response
- drug treatments that tend to be more focused on opiate use than on other types of drug use
- a harm reduction strategy that focuses on injecting and is perceived by some to lacking usefulness to non-injectors
- residential rehabilitation facilities that have often been found to be incapable of meeting diverse needs.

Further barriers to service take-up by adults from ethnic minority groups affected by either mental health or substance misuse issues are: that signposting information tends to be provided in English; most parenting programmes are evaluated with white and American samples; and no account is taken of potential differences in child-rearing and values (DfES 2006b).

In the Young Minds' study (Kurtz and others 2005), which was based on the views obtained from BME young people and staff working with them, they found the barriers to service take-up to be concerns among young people about:

- their previous experiences of discrimination and concerns about stigma
- their lack of a sense of inclusion in the local community
- the uncertain nature of the help they may have found, e.g. concerns about voluntary agencies closing due to lack of funds
- for those with uncertain legal status, how long they might be able to stay in the UK
- how to identify a mental health problem and what support would be available (felt by parents, too)

- 'going outside the family' to get help
- there being no interpreters available if they 'dropped in' for on-the-spot help
- staff in all services who had a poor awareness of their needs – conversely, young people greatly appreciated it when they found themselves 'finally understood' in specialist services
- a lack of choice in key members of staff, in terms of gender and cultural background, and a lack of younger staff from BME groups
- staff not always fully understanding the strong influence of parents' and communities' views and those of peer groups on the young people.

5. How can services support families more effectively at the practice level?

This chapter discusses some of the key factors in improving the effectiveness of support to families so as to enhance their, and their children's, resilience. It highlights approaches to overcoming the barriers to effective support at the practice level.

A wide variety of approaches to assessment are discussed.

At the practice level, it considers approaches to intervention.

The 'support to parents' and 'direct support to children' sections explore some of the factors that parents and children say are important for making services as useful and relevant to them as possible. Practice examples are given to illustrate an approach to the area of intervention under discussion.

Early intervention

It seems logical that the earlier people receive support, the more likely they are to overcome their difficulties. Better still, when difficulties seem likely to occur, the provision of services, support or the adoption of positive coping strategies can prevent problems arising, or at least from becoming overwhelming or entrenched. The case for early intervention and preventative practice is very strong, both morally and politically. Current policy drivers in all the relevant service areas point strongly towards early intervention as a priority in the future shape of services.

Practice example 1 is an example of how services in Brighton collaborated to produce a resource for secondary schools and provide support to enable appropriate early responses to young people affected by parental substance misuse.

Practice example 1: *The Hidden Ones* – Brighton and Hove

The Hidden Ones Communication Resource (2006) was produced in collaboration between Brighton and Hove Healthy Schools Team, Brighton Oasis Project, and Young Carers Project.

This resource takes the form of a communication pack. It comprises a range of information for secondary schools to use in conjunction with local agencies to support individual students in situations where parental substance misuse has been identified. The pack includes:

- guidance for schools on how to respond to children and young people identified as vulnerable because of parental substance misuse

---

- information to support an enhanced school policy in respect of children affected by parental substance misuse
- information on available support within secondary schools and within outside local agencies
- case study material to support appropriate practice responses to children and young people.

'Young Oasis' – a service for 5–18 year olds

'Young Oasis' is a service for children and young people affected by familial substance misuse and is based within The Brighton Oasis Project. It is a voluntary sector substance misuse service committed to preventing drug-related harm to women and children. 'Young Oasis' offers a variety of creative therapeutic interventions for children and young people affected by familial drug or alcohol misuse. These range from weekly one-to-one therapy sessions with a creative therapist , to a 'Young Women's Creative Therapy Group' run by qualified therapists in 12 week blocks, to holiday art groups during the school holidays with experienced group facilitators. 'Young Oasis' has also been delivering an outreach groupwork model within the local community. Children and young people are offered a 'First Meeting', from this consultation support is offered to suit an individual's needs.

For further information, please contact:
Jo Parker, 'Young Oasis', Brighton Oasis Project, 11 Richmond Place, Brighton BN2 9NA. Tel: 01273 696970 ext 203, or 0755 3360368

Key factors in promoting early intervention are accessible services with clear referral pathways and useful, relevant information provided to potential users and referrers, in locations where they are likely to access it. An agency seen to be promoting awareness and reducing stigma for people with mental health problems or substance misuse issues, could actively reach many potential service users who otherwise might have a negative view of the service. Also, making information about possible support services more readily available may mean more people, who might not otherwise have thought of or known about what might help them, accessing them earlier and probably gaining more from them than if referred when their problems are more extreme.

> One of the difficulties you'll have … is measuring demand because demand isn't always expressed in terms of 'I want this' because there isn't a sense of entitlement. People don't always ask for what they want because they don't know they could have it

(National Voluntary Organisation (DfES 2006b, p.33))

48

Voluntary versus compulsory support

Voluntary support is far more acceptable to families than compulsory intervention and more likely to lead to better outcomes. At the lower tiers of need, self-referrals are more likely, whereas at the higher tiers there are more professional referrals. Support at the higher tiers is more likely to involve a degree of compulsion, because by the time needs have reached this level, adverse impacts on children are so great that they have to be addressed. Compulsory interventions can still be effective, but close attention needs to be paid to helping people utilise and manage their experience of such interventions. Examples of this help include the following.

- Where parents are instructed to go on parenting courses – this is more likely to be effective if additional work takes place in advance of the courses to prepare parents for the group setting and ensure they are able to engage constructively and, not least, won't disrupt the group. Evidence suggests that such parents benefit from being mixed with parents who are receiving the support voluntarily (DfES 2006b).
- Where parents are referred for specialist assessments and interventions, such as residential assessments – again, adequate preparation for the experience and a view that there is real potential for it to be effective, rather than being 'a safe place to fail' (Hart and Powell 2006), can lead to more positive outcomes.
- Where families are receiving a service – skilful and purposeful interventions, which help support families to change by harnessing their strengths, are likely to be more productive than attempts to impose change.
- Where care proceedings have been initiated, in cases where parental substance misuse is a key element, and a Family Drug and Alcohol Court (FDAC) is in operation in that area, a specialist multi-disciplinary team of practitioners can assess, devise and coordinate an intervention with the family. The FDAC being piloted in the Inner London Proceedings Court (Harwin et al 2011) has shown promising results, with more parents engaging with services and more control of substance use by participating parents.

There will be times when compulsory intervention will mean children being removed permanently from their families because it has not been possible to ensure their safety at home. And sometimes this is for the best. Adoption and fostering can work well for some children. Forrester and Harwin (2006) found, in their study of cases within four London boroughs over two years, that many of the children who had been fostered or adopted in that time were showing better outcomes than those with similar family circumstances and experiences who were still at home.

However, even when such concrete and seemingly 'final decisions' have been made, such as applying for a care order and adoption, the needs of the family still need to be addressed. The impact on family members of what they have been through, the changes, transitions and arrangements for them to continue to see each other or to make sense of what has happened, need careful considered support.

Practice example 2 shows how a group parenting programme has engaged and supported women with mental health problems who have babies or young children.

Practice example 2: Mellow Parenting programme

The Mellow Parenting programme combines support for parents as individuals with direct work with them on their parenting. It developed from a recognition that parenting programmes based on social learning theory, though effective for many families in addressing children's behavioural problems, fail to engage about 50 per cent of families. Those who do not engage tend to be younger, less well educated and to have other personal and social needs including parental mental health problems. These are, of course, exactly the families who suffer the most health and social inequality. Other families who are in need of support for parenting may not meet the criteria of having a child with a behavioural problem. Around 10–20 per cent of mothers experience postnatal depression and their children are more likely to suffer psychological and behavioural problems themselves in later life and to do less well academically. For them, behaviourally based programmes are not the answer.

As an example, one single mother in her twenties had two children who were in kinship care because of neglect. She was homeless and had alcohol misuse problems. She had very poor literacy skills as she had more or less dropped out of school by the age of 10. Her family history was of a father who could only express any affection for his family when he was drunk; and a mother of extreme hostility and harshness, whose jingling bracelets approaching were a signal for the children to flee as they were sure to be given another beating. She attended the group regularly, began attending AA and asked to be rehoused. By the end of the fourteen weeks, she had the children back living with her although still under a supervision order. She was volunteering at the Family Centre and ran a ten-day cookery group for school age children single-handedly at the school holiday playscheme.

The programme works hard to recruit parents who, because of low self-esteem and mental health problems, find it hard to engage with services. By emphasising the positives in the interaction with their children, while acknowledging the difficulties, it invites them to find new ways of interacting with their children. The high attendance rate (80 per cent of parents attend 80 per cent of sessions) and good outcomes are a result of multiple factors, not least the respect for the individuality and value of each parent and child. Solutions are not prescribed and the support of the group is used to create a sense of empowerment for the members.

For further information contact:

info@mellowparenting.org
www.mellowparenting.org

Approaches to assessment

Most of the professionals reading this handbook are involved to some extent in undertaking assessments within their services – whether assessing potential users for eligibility for their service; tailoring the service appropriately; or by being a partner in a wider professional network and contributing through meetings, discussions and reports to an assessment being coordinated by someone else. Others work within lead agencies carrying out a formal assessment, such as a mental health assessment or an assessment under the *Framework for the Assessment of Children in Need and their Families* (Department of Health 2000).

More recently, the implementation of the Common Assessment Framework following the Children Act 2004 means that an even greater variety of relevant professionals are involved in assessments. Assessments should always be based on clear and rigorous analysis of information about the family in a way that makes the process transparent and explicable to a broad audience. The issue of analysis within assessments is an important one though it is not always a straightforward process, since weighing up complex issues necessarily involves deploying a range of analytical and intuitive processes, skills and knowledge.

From 2003 to 2005, the National Children's Bureau project *Putting Analysis into Assessment* explored how practitioners could be supported in improving the analytical element of assessment by introducing different tools and approaches. These are described in detail in Dalzell and Sawyer (2007), but some of the points are highlighted below.

Assessment as intervention

There is a thin line between assessment and intervention and often the distinction is false or over-simplistic. Assessments are not simply about matching service users to services; about gate-keeping resources; or investigating deficits in family functioning. Done well, assessments can and should increase service users' self-knowledge, and improve their desire to make changes and be family-friendly. Also, when undertaken reflectively, assessments should lead to professionals identifying their own needs for additional skills or training and, through identifying and recording any unmet service user needs, helping agencies to learn about the need for the creation of additional services and opportunities (Hamer 2005).

There is a particular challenge for those undertaking child protection investigations or core assessments to engage families in the process in a way that is beneficial to them. If some level of partnership or collaboration between worker and service user can be established early on, this can make all the difference to the direction that family circumstances and intervention take later on. Turnell and Edwards (1999) argue that even child protection investigations can be therapeutic, in that they can help develop a family's understanding of the issues affecting them and offer support and education, with interventions being 'the icing on the cake'. They see the relationship between professional and service user as having the potential to be the principal vehicle for change.

Values and reflectivity

It is essential that those undertaking assessments are able to recognise the impact of their feelings and values on their assessment and interactions with families.

Forrester (2004) stresses the importance of this in relation to substance misuse because it is such a value-laden subject. All individual professionals will have some preconceptions, concerns, stereotypes or experience (personal or professional) of substance or alcohol use that affect their responses to it. Preconceptions could influence one in favour of either over-zealous interventions or naïve and over-optimistic inaction. This can also be said of mental ill health, where there are the dangers of over-reacting due to fear and misunderstanding, reinforced by frequent media portrayal of 'dangerousness'. Conversely, feeling great sympathy for people in distress and wanting to help or prove to them that you are not there to make things worse, can make it harder to respond quickly and appropriately if they are becoming unable to meet their children's needs.

In social research, a 'cultural review' checklist is sometimes used (devised by McCracken (1988)) at the outset of the work. Holland (2004) adapted the original checklist for social work use. Undertaking the review involves asking oneself questions at the outset of work or on receipt of referral information, such as:

- What do I know about individuals with these life experiences?
- Where does my knowledge come from?
- What prejudices may I hold (positive or negative)?
- What might surprise me and why would it be a surprise?
- How might I/the assessment and my agency be perceived by this family?
- What agency norms and practices do I take with me on an assessment (e.g. awareness of risk, thresholds of 'good enough parenting', resource restrictions)?

This approach helps bring preconceived ideas or values into consciousness, in order to help minimise their potential adverse impact on the integrity of an assessment.

Hypothesising

There is a tendency for first impressions to last and for human beings to seek out and notice information that supports their original ideas (Scott 1998, Sheldon 1987). Information that is contrary to strongly held views or ideas is more easily dismissed or even goes unnoticed. Once again, social research methods can assist here. Holland (2004) discusses the importance of 'hypothesising' at the outset and (at staged intervals) throughout assessments. A hypothesis is a proposed explanation for something; so in a family support context, a hypothesis is a way of understanding a family situation. For example, if a child is frequently late for school or is increasingly tired and withdrawn there could be a range of reasons for this, including the following.

- It may be a result of increased parental stress whereby the child is not receiving the usual level of support with getting up and ready for school.
- It could be that the child is anxious about a school matter.
- It could be they are worried about a move to secondary school and not sleeping as a result.
- The child may have a substance misuse problem.

The presence of different factors (known about by professionals) will all influence which hypothesis or hypotheses are held at different stages.

This process of generating ideas about family situations usually occurs almost naturally. However, if left at this, the chances are that only two or three ideas will be generated and the natural human tendency to find information that supports these ideas will kick in. Raynes (Calder and Hackett 2003) suggests the need to generate as many hypotheses early on as possible and Holland (2004) suggests then actively seeking to disprove each one, identifying information that confirms or disproves them until one or two strong explanations emerge that are well supported.

Needs and outcome focus

Assessments are most likely to be helpful if they are focused on needs and outcomes. There can be a tendency to jump to considering services too early on. For example if in response to the question What might be the needs for this child/family?, the response includes things such as:

- speech therapy
- further assessment by [some specialist agency]
- counselling
- behavioural management support or respite care

then the question has not been answered. These are all services and, whilst telling us what possible options there are for meeting needs, the actual needs are still unknown.

By stepping back and considering what the needs might be (that the above options could possibly meet), we may come up with some of the following.

- The child needs to develop their verbal or communication skills to enable them to interact more with their peers.
- A parent needs support in addressing their alcohol dependence.
- A parent needs help in stabilising their severe mood swings or anxiety.
- An adolescent needs support with a bereavement.
- A parent needs help in setting boundaries for their child.
- A parent needs a break from caring for their disabled child so that they can give some one-to-one attention to their non-disabled child.

It is this latter list of needs that should be the starting point, with services being considered later down the line.

Once the needs of family members are identified, then 'outcomes' can be considered. We can ask, if the child's need were met – how would we know? What would this look like? It may be thought that if the child starts speaking more in class and interacting more confidently with their peers, we can see that as a concrete outcome of the need being met. Only then, when we have identified needs and what the outcome of them being met would involve, is it appropriate to consider what things might individually or collectively help move towards that outcome.

There is usually more than one approach to meeting the same need. If needs are the starting point for intervention rather than services, then if one service makes a family wary or adds to their stress, another form of intervention can be considered that may be more acceptable and useful to the family. This approach fits well with the use of the Common Assessment Framework and the *Framework for Assessment of Children in Need and their Families* (Department of Health 2000) and is discussed more fully in Dalzell and Sawyer (2011).

Resilience/vulnerability matrix

The resilience/vulnerability matrix provides a framework for weighing up factors that create adversity in children's lives and increase their vulnerability alongside those factors that research has shown can contribute to increased resilience. It is particularly appropriate for assessment where parents have mental health and substance misuse problems given the multi-faceted nature of these difficulties.

Using the resilience/vulnerability matrix

Completion of the matrix requires the practitioner to have a working knowledge of resilience theory and the factors that contribute to the different axes of the matrix. A good starting point would be to read Daniel, Wassell and Gilligan (2010) *Child Development for Child Care and Protection Workers* (chapters 4 and 5).

Sufficient information will need to have been accumulated from assessment or other interaction with a child, their carers, family and involved professionals. Each axis of the matrix contains a scale from 0 to 10, with 0 being an absence of factors contributing to that domain of the matrix and 10 being the highest incidence of contributory factors.

Taking each axis in turn, the information that has been gathered is scored on the 0–10 scale. For example, for a child with a secure attachment, good problem-solving skills, popular with peers, high IQ and doing well at school this would most likely lead to a high score on the **resilience** axis of the matrix. If, however, that child has been self-harming for some time and this is becoming more severe over time, and they are developing anxiety problems that are interfering with their day to day life, a score to reflect this would be placed on the **vulnerability** axis. If the same young person is living in a family situation with domestic abuse, parental mental ill health and financial insecurity this would indicate a significant score on the **adversity** axis, but if they also have good relationships with teachers and other adults and made good use of support and advice offered from the school counsellor this would be noted on the **protective environment** axis. The matrix is most useful when used as an interactive tool with children and young people as active agents in the process.

There are no right and wrong answers and the scoring will be a matter of professional judgement, indeed whenever we use this tool in training there are vigorous debates as to the impact, harmful or beneficial of various factors in children's lives. The completion of the matrix only represents the understanding of the child's situation at that time and by those involved in constructing it. It will be informed by theory, research, practice wisdom, local knowledge and information gleaned from a range of sources, including the child themselves. The process of considering and plotting the information is in itself a useful process and requires thoughtfulness and possibly debate if being done with others, but there is another stage that can create a powerful visual map. Once all of the axes have been considered and plotted, the points can be joined with a drawn line to create a shape that will be spread across the four domains (located more within some than others). This visual map can help in assessment and planning by providing a snapshot, but can also be useful for recording progress if completed at various intervals.

Where the shape sits predominantly in the top right-hand quadrant of the two axes this suggest that the child is both resilient and protected and more likely to be able to recover from any difficulties they face. This is the safest area for children to be and universal services can support and build on these positive factors.

Where the shape sits predominantly in the lower right quadrant this indicates that the child is protected, but for whatever reason also vulnerable. This will mean that the planning for this child should focus on maintaining the support whilst building up their resilience.

Where the shape sits predominantly in the top left quadrant, this indicates a child who exhibits signs of resilience whilst remaining in adverse circumstances. These are the children that targeted and specialist services should be working with to increase the level of protection, in partnership with the child and their family, whether by raising them from poverty or taking action to safeguard against abuse. One criticism of this model is that resilient children in risky situations may be ignored as relatively safe. It is crucial to recognise that no matter how resilient children may be, there will be times when the risks are too severe to ignore and the presence of resilience factors should never be an excuse for lack of attention or inaction.

If the shape sits predominantly in the lower left corner of the graph it indicates the most vulnerable child who does not have resilience or factors within their environment to provide protection. This child will need intensive specialist intervention. As well as identifying the associated risk this model allows us to develop care plans in two directions – to increase the level of protection and to improve children's resilience, improving the chances of reducing risk.

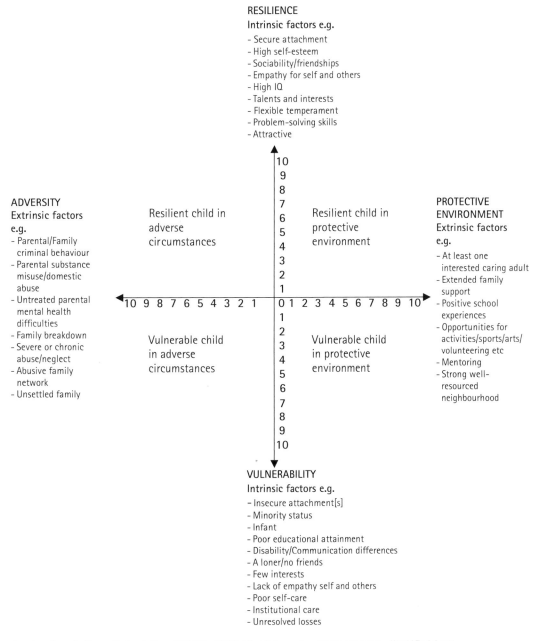

RESILIENCE
Intrinsic factors e.g.
- Secure attachment
- High self-esteem
- Sociability/friendships
- Empathy for self and others
- High IQ
- Talents and interests
- Flexible temperament
- Problem-solving skills
- Attractive

ADVERSITY
Extrinsic factors e.g.
- Parental/Family criminal behaviour
- Parental substance misuse/domestic abuse
- Untreated parental mental health difficulties
- Family breakdown
- Severe or chronic abuse/neglect
- Abusive family network
- Unsettled family

Resilient child in adverse circumstances

Resilient child in protective environment

PROTECTIVE ENVIRONMENT
Extrinsic factors e.g.
- At least one interested caring adult
- Extended family support
- Positive school experiences
- Opportunities for activities/sports/arts/ volunteering etc
- Mentoring
- Strong well-resourced neighbourhood

Vulnerable child in adverse circumstances

Vulnerable child in protective environment

VULNERABILITY
Intrinsic factors e.g.
- Insecure attachment[s]
- Minority status
- Infant
- Poor educational attainment
- Disability/Communication differences
- A loner/no friends
- Few interests
- Lack of empathy self and others
- Poor self-care
- Institutional care
- Unresolved losses

Based on figure in Horwarth, J and others (2000) The Child's World: Assessing children in need – World Training & Development Pack. London: NSPCC

Figure 2: Resilience/vulnerability matrix

Representing children's views and needs in assessments

Some professionals who work directly with children as a matter of course, providing specialist or universal services directly to them, are particularly skilled in recognising and describing children's needs and feelings. Others whose role is wider – either working with whole families or with individual parents or carers – may need support in interpreting or understanding children's experience.

For those professionals such as social workers who need to try and establish children's needs, views and wishes, they may find consulting with a range of people who know the child, observing the child in a range of settings and finding out about others' observations in a variety of settings over time helpful. Disabled children's views and perspectives are particularly poorly represented in assessments, as practitioners often lack the confidence, skills and creativity to access their feelings and views. Drawing on all possible resources, creative communication techniques and using equipment or facilitators where appropriate, in addition to allowing sufficient time to enable children to contribute to assessment, are essential.

In reality, the information and knowledge about children's views and wishes will often be partial, so it is important to acknowledge gaps and limitations in our understanding so that we don't misrepresent children through assumptions or partial information.

Kroll and Taylor 2003 suggest that 'keeping the child in mind' in assessments involves asking 'What is this child experiencing:

- when they wake up?
- at school?
- in the evening?
- during the night?
- when parents are intoxicated?
- when parents are unwell?
- when parents are sober?'

As well as asking 'What has this child experienced in past months and what will they experience in the months and years to come?'

Placing knowledge in context

The information available to those carrying out assessments will usually be partial, hence the importance of putting knowledge and information into context within assessment reports or when communicating about the family situation. Assessments can sometimes be over-reliant on short-term observations, focusing on acute episodes rather than everyday life (Aldridge 1999). Clearly identifying the extent of knowledge of the family that is available, and being explicit about gaps in knowledge, is the only way to reduce the misrepresentation that can occur.

Also, showing awareness and sensitivity about the stress generated by the assessment process itself (or by the search for support, or even receiving the support itself), will help place family reactions to this stress into context. Turnell and Edwards (1999) give the following example to illustrate this. If a parent leaves a meeting early in frustration, they can all too easily be labelled 'uncooperative' when in fact they had a terrible week, were being asked questions they had been asked before and thought that professionals had 'already made up their minds'.

Turnell and Edwards stress the need to 'search for detail': to explore all positive and negative factors from sources inside and outside the family. This, they argue, will make it more possible to 'identify antecedents, consequences, patterns, feelings and opportunities for change' (Turnell and Edwards 1999).

Analysing the impact of specific issues

Most of the points made so far in relation to assessments apply to assessments of family members affected by parental mental health problems and/or substance misuse. All assessments should focus on the wide-ranging needs and experiences of families. Whilst this broad focus is right and helpful, and indeed parents have often given feedback that they want professionals to see their lives as a whole and not to attribute all their difficulties to mental health or substance problems (Tunnard 2002a and 2004), there is still a place for specific attention to issues such as the impact of substance use, mental health, and domestic violence.

In each case, appropriate assessment of risk and protective factors should be considered and offered. In the following two sections, some of the areas for specific consideration in these circumstances are highlighted.

When it comes to decision making, the key questions that arise from the models that follow are: What needs to change to protect the child now or minimise the future impact of these problems on them? and How can this be achieved? In thinking about the latter, the professional needs to consider the questions:

- Can resilience factors be bolstered?
- Can risks be reduced through support to the family?
- What are the wishes and feelings of the child?
- What timescales are appropriate to the child's needs?
- How does the likelihood of plans succeeding weigh against the potential impact of failure?
- If a child cannot be cared for by their family how can future relationships be supported?

Substance misuse

A range of helpful models has been developed to assist practitioners in focusing their assessment of the impact of parental substance misuse on children.

For example Hart and Powell (2006) have devised a very helpful Model for Assessment of Parental Drug Use, which overlays the *Framework for Assessment of Children in Need and their Families* with particular questions of pertinence for children of drug-using parents (see Appendix 3).

Professional responses need to be based on assessment and analysis of the specific needs of individual children and families; the risks present for them; the impact of these risks; and the presence of protective factors, parental motivation and capacity to change. Those undertaking assessments need to be mindful of the impact their own values and expectations, and those of others, could potentially have on the assessment and to guard against this.

Short-term risks of immediate harm need to be assessed along with those of longer-term risks to give the cumulative impact on the child or young person's emotional and behavioural well-being. It is also essential to consider how other issues and factors that are present but not directly related to substance misuse (such as family conflict or a learning disability) are impacting on the child and affecting their circumstances.

Forrester (2004, Chapter 10) puts forward the following Four Assessment Principles to assist in focusing assessments of children's needs when there is parental substance misuse.

Four Assessment Principles

1   Maintain a focus on the child. Collecting information on the pattern of drug use is of limited utility in making an assessment if all the other variables are not focused on. How does the substance use impact on the child? How is the child progressing and understanding any reasons for the difficulties they may have?

2   Adults' management of their own life can be a good indicator of their ability to look after a child (the measure being whether the parent is causing themselves harm through a failure to manage their own lives).

3   Past behaviour is the best predictor of future behaviour. A good chronology and full social history, which is best completed by involving the parent and young person (if appropriate), can greatly assist this.

4   A variety of sources should be used for information. This includes different agencies along with wider family, such as grandparents, as valuable sources of information and support.

(Adapted from Donald Forrester's work in Phillips (2004) *Children Exposed to Parental Substance Misuse: Implications for family placement*, BAAF, pp.172–4)

The model in Figure 3 utilises and adapts models produced by Forrester (2004) and Hart and Powell (2006) to highlight the risk and protective factors that need to be weighed up when considering the impact of substance misuse on children and their families.

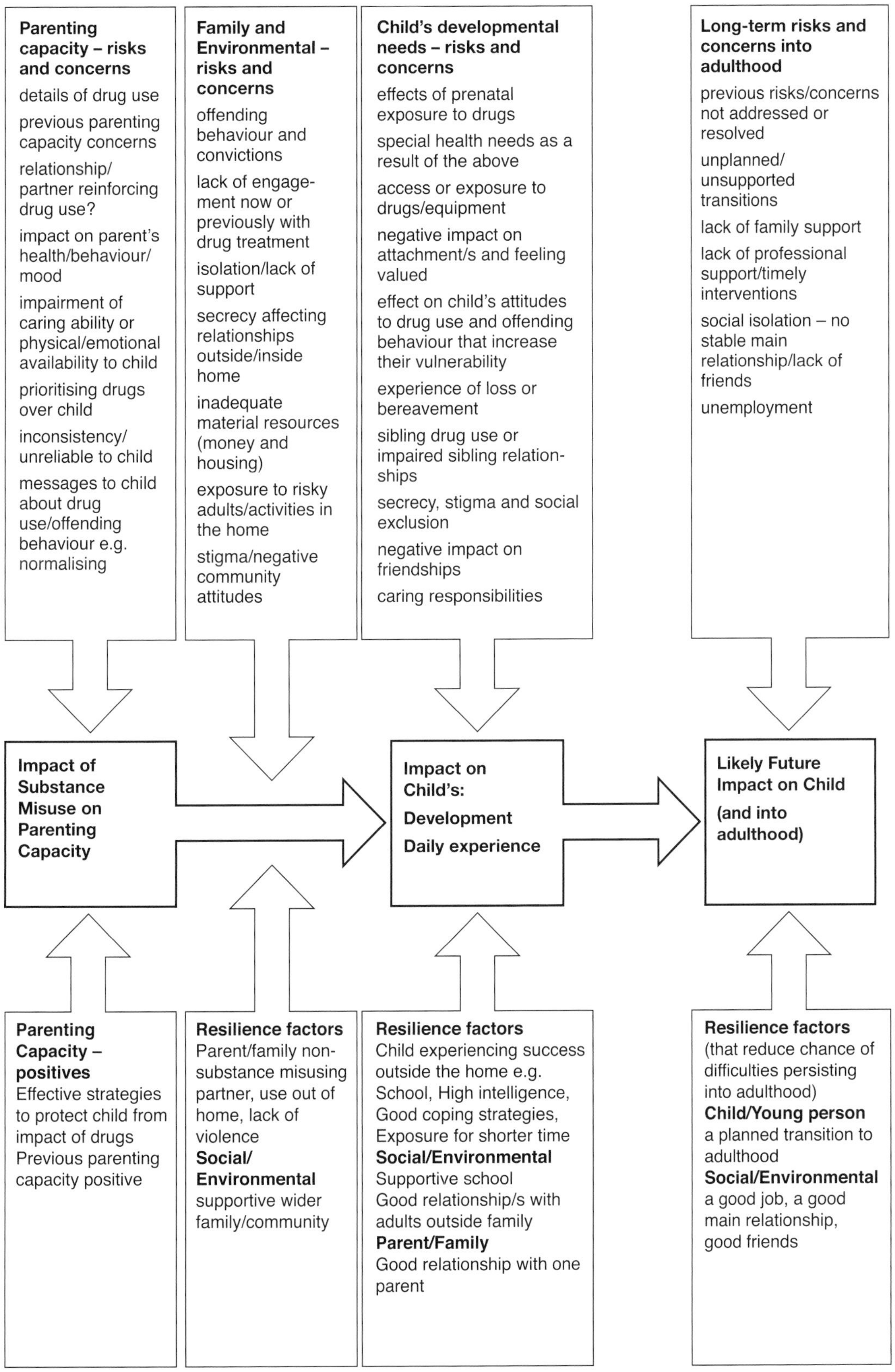

Parenting capacity – risks and concerns

details of drug use

previous parenting capacity concerns

relationship/ partner reinforcing drug use?

impact on parent's health/behaviour/ mood

impairment of caring ability or physical/emotional availability to child

prioritising drugs over child

inconsistency/ unreliable to child

messages to child about drug use/offending behaviour e.g. normalising

Family and Environmental – risks and concerns

offending behaviour and convictions

lack of engage- ment now or previously with drug treatment

isolation/lack of support

secrecy affecting relationships outside/inside home

inadequate material resources (money and housing)

exposure to risky adults/activities in the home

stigma/negative community attitudes

Child's developmental needs – risks and concerns

effects of prenatal exposure to drugs

special health needs as a result of the above

access or exposure to drugs/equipment

negative impact on attachment/s and feeling valued

effect on child's attitudes to drug use and offending behaviour that increase their vulnerability

experience of loss or bereavement

sibling drug use or impaired sibling relation- ships

secrecy, stigma and social exclusion

negative impact on friendships

caring responsibilities

Long-term risks and concerns into adulthood

previous risks/concerns not addressed or resolved

unplanned/ unsupported transitions

lack of family support

lack of professional support/timely interventions

social isolation – no stable main relationship/lack of friends

unemployment

Impact of Substance Misuse on Parenting Capacity

Impact on Child's:
Development
Daily experience

Likely Future Impact on Child
(and into adulthood)

Parenting Capacity – positives
Effective strategies to protect child from impact of drugs
Previous parenting capacity positive

Resilience factors
Parent/family non- substance misusing partner, use out of home, lack of violence
Social/ Environmental
supportive wider family/community

Resilience factors
Child experiencing success outside the home e.g. School, High intelligence, Good coping strategies, Exposure for shorter time
Social/Environmental
Supportive school
Good relationship/s with adults outside family
Parent/Family
Good relationship with one parent

Resilience factors
(that reduce chance of difficulties persisting into adulthood)
Child/Young person
a planned transition to adulthood
Social/Environmental
a good job, a good main relationship, good friends

Figure 3: Links in a chain

Harbin and Murphy (2000) put forward the model in Figure 4. Where possible, this should be considered jointly by substance misuse and child and family practitioners so as to optimise the information available and the understanding of practitioners of the family circumstances.

The first stage involves gaining an understanding of the nature of substance use, including its impact on the lifestyle of the parent and their relationship to the substance or its 'meaning' for them. The second stage considers both the parent's own experience of being parented, their attitudes and expectations about their own parenting role and the impact of their substance use (or withdrawal) on their parenting. The third stage considers the impact these factors have on the child and any needs they have arising from this. The last stage involves consideration of the level of child-care demand on the parent, which will be influenced by the age, developmental stage and number of children, as well as the support available from other adults.

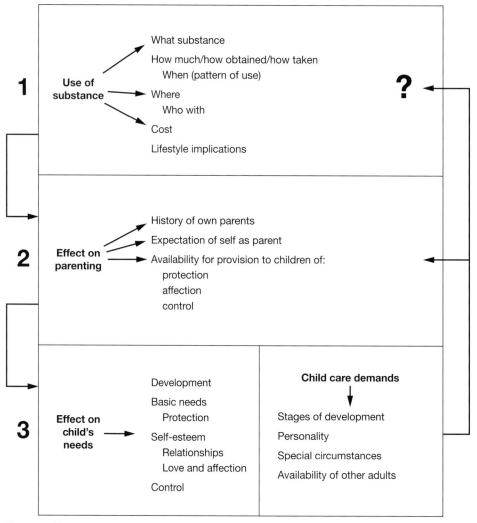

Figure 4: The assessment process

There can be a tendency for children's practitioners (from non-drug-specialist services) to push for total abstinence from parental drug use. This is not always necessary or realistic and an emphasis on total change can make it harder for parents to make smaller, more realistic changes. Stabilising drug use and a harm-minimisation approach can be more realistic and helpful. Of course where service users desire abstinence, their efforts to achieve it should be supported, with awareness that the stress within the family may initially increase as a result. After all, substance use can be seen as a 'coping strategy' or, for some, as a form of 'self-medication' which will need replacing with alternative ways of coping.

An increased understanding of the nature of substance addiction and the process of change (or the Cycle of Change Model developed by Prochaska and others (1994)) might help relevant professionals to better support such change, at a pace that is right for, and driven by, service users. Within this model there is an acceptance that change is not easy and that people may need repeated opportunities to achieve the desired objective. The nature of the intervention should be determined by, and appropriate to, the stage in the cycle at which the person seems to be.

Cycle of Change Model

1 **Pre-contemplation**
   The person sees no reason to change their behaviour – whatever the advice offered.

2 **Contemplation**
   The person considers making a change at some point in the future, but is still unsure about making a firm commitment to it.

3 **Preparation**
   A decision to change is taken, the person takes some personal responsibility for the desired changes and starts planning to take action.

4 **Action**
   The person actively pursues the desired change. Observable effort is made to break with old habits or to develop a new, more positive, one.

5 **Maintenance**
   The desired change has been achieved, and lasted for some time. The main task at this stage is to prevent oneself from slipping back into old habits (relapse prevention).

(Adapted from Prochaska and others 1994)

The guilt, shame and remorse that many parents feel is hard to face (Kroll and Taylor 2003) and needs to be considered sensitively within the approach taken to assessment.

Many parents are strongly motivated by wanting to put things right for their children. Becoming a parent or realising the impact the addiction has on parenting can be strong motivators for change; as can, in some circumstances, the reality of children potentially being separated from parents (Bates and others 1999). Assessments need to search for strengths and scope for change. Harnessing the motivation of parents is key to the success of interventions.

Mental health

In supporting families affected by parental mental health issues it is important to establish patterns that occur, in order to find ways of identifying early on when mental health is deteriorating or relapse is occurring. Establishing potential arrangements for early identification, ongoing monitoring and access to support and intervention when necessary is ideal, but requires proactive and flexible services.

The following is a possible framework to guide the assessment process.

The following provides a list of dimensions to be explored in assessments of families affected by parental mental health problems. This is taken from Gopfert and others (2004).

Dimensions of parenting formulation

Focus on the role of parent – this includes assessing parenting capacity in line with the Assessment Framework headings. It also includes ensuring there is consideration of 'age appropriate understanding and expectations of child, including capacity to talk with child about parent's mental illness' and any evidence of 'role reversal'.

Focus on role of child – this includes considering the child's developmental needs within the Assessment Framework; their attachment status; any unusual, 'non-childlike' behaviour, including involvement in parent's symptoms or substance misuse and 'parentification'; and what protective factors are present.

Focus on the impact of mental illness on the role of parent – this includes considering the parent's:

- sense of responsibility for self, child and family
- capacity to acknowledge risks to child
- level of disturbance, instability and violent tendencies (impulse control)
- behaviour and psychiatric symptoms where they directly affect parenting capacity, including alcohol/substance misuse
- level of commitment to child
- motivation for change, including past history
- capacity to reflect
- attitude to social norms/relationship to society
- attitude to professionals; use of help and clinical interventions.

Focus on the role of 'well'/other parent (if relevant) – this includes considering the other parent's:

- commitment to maintaining the family or commitment to the relationship with the child
- capacity to be available/to intervene on the child's behalf, if and when necessary
- relationship to the child
- attitude to the illness of their partner
- health and emotional resources.

Focus on role of spouse/partner (if relevant) – this includes considering the extent to which there is any:

- history of violence/spouse abuse
- capacity to work together as parents

- patterns, style and intensity of marital conflict
- ability to communicate.

Focus on context and extended family – this includes considering the following factors:

- access to relationship with an adult who is committed to providing support and care for child and/or parent
- degree and patterns of support from extended family, directly to child as well as to parent
- parent's relationship to own parents
- quality of non-family network
- financial/housing status
- environmental stress/life events/current stressors.

Approaches to intervention

The needs and welfare of the child must remain firmly in focus throughout any work with children and families. Finely balanced judgements and decisions will have to be made. Work must be continuously and systematically reviewed to guard against the twin perils of *either* 'drift/distraction' on to the specific needs of adults *or* precipitate reactive practice. For the sake of the children involved, attempts to facilitate change should not be persisted in where parental resistance to it is such that it becomes clear families are unlikely or unwilling to change. In such circumstances, professionals must intervene to protect the child's welfare. The following are some considerations to help guide practice in an area where maintaining clarity and focus can be a challenge.

Timing

Timing is very important in harnessing motivation and delays can mean it is lost. The 'window of opportunity' that is presented in a crisis (when people's normal coping mechanisms break down) is thought to last around 4–6 weeks (Roberts 1990).

There is a need to consider each party's own needs in relation to timescales. This often results in tensions because:

> *the developing nature of a young child demands a different framework of time to the needs of a chronically ill parent or the bureaucratic needs of the court*

> (Gopfert and others 2004, p.94)

This involves weighing up the developmental needs of a child against probable 'recovery' time for parents.

Strength and goal focus

Solution focused, systemic interventions, in which it is assumed as a starting point that parents probably want the best for their children and will utilise services if offered appropriately, tend to be helpful. Studies have previously reported on parents feeling that they are 'seen as a case' during assessments and there being an emphasis on deficits and weaknesses. They often describe a stream of professionals focusing on weakness, which over time undermines their sense of their own abilities (Turnell and Edwards 1999). In *Signs of Safety: A solution and safety-orientated approach to child protection*, Turnell and Edwards argue that there is only limited usefulness in assessments, which focus entirely on deficits (for example: Which needs aren't met? Which risks are present?). They argue that a greater focus on strengths and a better consideration of the goals and values of parents makes true partnership and collaboration far more likely.

Questions regarding strengths can generate useful information for families and professionals. If someone is unable to see any strengths or positives this, in itself, could provide useful information.

In the *Signs of Safety* approach, the authors suggest the following ways of eliciting information about strengths.

- Use exception questions, such as 'Tell me about times when you/the parent has been managing well?' The question is based on assumptions that the problem isn't happening constantly and that the parent probably manages the problem some of the time. The answers elicited from questions such as this can uncover safe, constructive behaviours.
- Ensure that the detail of the 'exception' is explored, the *how, when, where and what.*
- Explore, knowing that it's possible, how confident the person is in their ability to repeat the exception.

Turnell and Edwards stress that this does involve a shift in conversation, so they recommend ensuring the 'problem' has been fully acknowledged before exploring exceptions; and to ask the question in three ways before moving on, not to expect people to be able to change their focus from the problem at the first time of asking.

Some participants on the Building Resilience project discussed how much easier it is to bring up and engage in discussions about concerns and problems when an atmosphere of looking at positives has already been established. A strengths-based approach is not about just staying with what is comfortable, but is about there being more balance and engagement.

Another way of harnessing existing strengths and potential for change is through identifying the goals of service users. An explicit emphasis on goals is another feature of solution-focused approaches and the *Signs of Safety* model.

> *Intake is a process of setting clear goal posts so that everybody knows what behaviour is expected and can clearly see when it has been achieved*

> (Hamer 2005, p.14)

If goals are coming primarily from professionals, it can be more helpful for them to focus on 'presence rather than absence', for example telling a parent they need to be in earshot and eyesight of the baby at all times rather than telling them to stop leaving the child unattended or unsupervised (Turnell and Edwards 1999). Also, when setting goals with (and ideally driven by) family members, these goals need to have clearly specified outcomes and be broken down into manageable steps. Achievable measures of success defined by parents are better than over-optimistic expectations. This helps to ensure that parents are not set up to fail. For example, in some cases substance use reduction or control is a more realistic goal than abstinence and can significantly increase family stability.

Within Brief Therapy approaches, change is viewed as continuous; so one change will inevitably lead to another (Cade and O'Hanlon 1993). Focusing on specific small changes can lead to a sense of achievement, increased confidence and readiness for more, whereas big goals can be frustrating and undermine confidence.

Strengths and values cards (see Practice example 3) are one approach to eliciting information from families about what things are important to them and what their values and goals are.

Practice example 3 shows how a family drug and alcohol service focuses on strengths and goals to encourage better outcomes for families.

Practice example 3: CASA Family Service, London

Since July 2006, CASA Family Service has been offering an accessible therapeutic service to families affected by parental use of alcohol or other drugs. It helps families to build on their strengths and develop ways of minimising harm, caused by parental use of alcohol or other drugs, to family members and particularly to children and young people.

Background

CASA Family Service has grown out of the work of CASA, a voluntary sector alcohol and drug service for adults based in North London. Over a number of years, CASA has developed services for parents and carers and was in a good position to develop a family service when the opportunity arose via commissioning from the local Drug and Alcohol Action Team (DAAT) in the London Borough of Islington.

This commissioning arrangement with the DAAT has positioned the service within an overall strategy of Hidden Harm services for children, young people and their families within the local borough of Islington – thus ensuring good multi-agency links across statutory and voluntary sector adult and children's services from the outset.

Practice approach

The work with families, and with the professional networks around them, aims to help parents and carers build up patterns of protective parenting and thereby increase the resilience of children and young people. After initial sessions with parents or carers on their own, parents and children are invited to attend weekly family sessions together, during which a semi-structured model of intervention is followed. The model was developed by Wendy Robinson as a practice approach called Child-Focused Family Intervention.

Family values and strengths cards

An integral part of this approach is the use of card-sort exercises to start therapeutic conversations with families in the first few sessions. These are engaging and accessible to children of all ages as well as to adults; and offer families the space to talk more readily about their family circumstances and personal views. The card-sort exercises are particularly designed to invite families to talk about what matters most to them in their family life; which of these things get affected by difficulties such as parental use of alcohol or drugs; and what strengths and resources they have to build on. Often families find that this process allows them to identify more clearly how they want family life to be and how it currently is, or has been, affected by parental use of alcohol or drugs. This process can lead to a strong sense of motivation to change while also encouraging a family's sense of confidence to achieve manageable change. Within this strengths-based approach, CASA particularly work with families to identify parenting strengths, in order to create a safer and more secure family environment.

Following the card-sort exercises, families are enabled to identify manageable goals for change in their work with the service – primarily in relation to alcohol or other drug use, parenting, and children's needs. These goals are shared with referrers where appropriate, and are reviewed with the family at regular intervals. In addition to family sessions, there is direct work with children or parents and carers on an individual basis; interventions are tailored to the particular needs and choices of each family.

Collaborative working with support networks

CASA have found it helpful to take a proactive and collaborative stance with families and the professional networks with which they often engage. In order to work with the whole system of support around family members, CASA aims to find a balance between prioritising client confidentiality within its therapeutic work with making clear agreements about sharing information with other professionals when this is supportive to family members.

Ben Kandelaars
CASA Family Service Manager
86 Durham Road
London
N7 7DU
020 7561 7490
Email: ben.kandelaars@casa.org.uk

Working with resistance

Forms of resistance – such as denial and minimisation of problems – are often associated with addiction but also apply to other problems that are too difficult to face or with which people feel immobilised. Working with resistance is very challenging and many professionals have little training or preparation in responding to this constructively.

Approaches that involve challenging and confronting people or 'trying to make them see or admit' to the extent of their problems, tend to increase the likelihood of people feeling defensive or feeling the need to hide things even more and of them withdrawing. Statutory children and families services often use such approaches when there are child protection concerns. Practitioners in such services, and in fact all practitioners trying to engage with people who they feel are resistant, should consider critically the extent to which their practices are unintentionally reinforcing such denial.

Miller and Rollnick (2002) argue that good empathic listening, which is at the heart of their Motivational Interviewing approach, is far more productive.

There is strong evidence that Motivational Interviewing works in brief interventions (Treasure 2004, and see also www.rcpsych.ac.uk). In many controlled trials, the approach has been found to be almost always effective; and it has been effective in relation to alcohol and substance misuse, medication compliance, dual diagnosis, mental illness treatment and eating disorders.

The principles of the approach are broadly compatible with core social work values. It is client centred; empathic; and involves reducing resistance and collaborating with service users towards change. It does this through:

- understanding
- giving choice and control
- questioning in a curious, open, empathic way and using 'change talk'.

Miller and Rollnick set out the following components of the approach and some general principles (Miller and Rollnick 2002, p.34).

The Motivational Interviewing (MI) approach

There are three key components of the MI approach: collaboration, evocation and autonomy.

Collaboration – involves counsellor and client working together towards goals that emerge from their collaboration. It requires the counsellor/interviewer to be aware of the attitudes and goals that they themselves bring to the interpersonal relationship. It also involves the creation of a positive atmosphere 'conducive to change'.

Evocation – involves 'drawing out' (like water from a well) the intrinsic motivation from the person – not 'imparting'.

Autonomy – refers to the fact that the responsibility for change must lie with the client. When MI is done properly, it's the client not the counsellor who presents the arguments for change.

The four general principles of the MI approach are as follows.

1   **Express empathy** – as it is fundamental to effectiveness (as described by Carl Rogers, 1962); and the 'acceptance' of people 'as they are' is crucial and seems to free people up to change. Conversely, family therapists use a term – 'ironic process' – where an action causes the response it is designed to prevent, for example saying 'you have to change' immobilises people. Ambivalence is accepted as a normal part of human experience and not pathology.

2   **Develop discrepancy** – as MI is intentionally directive (unlike person-centred counselling). The goal is to amplify the discrepancy between the person's behaviour and their goals or values.

3   **Roll with resistance** – otherwise, if the counsellor advocates change and the client argues against it, it is counter-productive and may even push the client further in the opposite direction. In MI, the counsellor doesn't 'oppose resistance, but rolls or flows with it' and resistance is a signal to shift approach. New perspectives are invited (from the client by turning questions or problems back on the person) and not imposed.

4   **Support self-efficacy** – as this term refers to a person's belief in his or her ability to succeed with something and is an important part of motivation. A counsellor's belief in a client's ability to change can create a self-fulfilling prophecy. The authors raise some concerns with the notion of 'resistance', which implies one person is resistant (they think it is more relational than that). 'Client resistance behaviour' is seen as 'a signal of dissonance within the relationship'.

Forrester argues that social workers (and others) would benefit from applying the principles of an MI approach in their work. Through research, Forrester found that for some practitioners, basic training in the approach improved listening skills, resulted in a less confrontational style, a reduced tendency to impose a social work agenda and, as a result, an increased ability to engage constructively with service users (Forrester 2004, Forrester and others 2008).

The term Motivational Interviewing (MI) strictly applies to the use of the technique by fully trained clinicians. However, others can draw on some of the methods, and most importantly the underlying principles, and this can benefit their approach. Substance-misuse professionals are commonly trained in the approach.

'Think family'

Much has been said already about the need for professionals, both individually and collectively, to widen their thinking – particularly if they are from a service that is primarily set up for individual family members – to include the families of which those members are a part. In June 2007, the then Labour government published *Reaching Out: Think family – Analysis and themes from the Families At Risk Review* (Cabinet Office, Social Exclusion Task Force). This examined the challenges of engaging with, and supporting, families with multiple problems who remain in poverty with complex needs and multiple, often interacting, problems. It argued that if were to really reach out to these families and enable them to overcome their problems, we had to develop the capacity of services to 'think family'. The current coalition government has signalled a clear intention to continue with this focus on complex families. On 15 December 2011 the prime minister announced plans and a £450m fund to support robust engagement aimed at turning around the lives of 120,000 of those he described as some of the country's most 'troubled families'. Central to the scheme, which bears some resemblance to the previous government's Family Intervention Projects, is a dedicated worker to coordinate and work with the family to tackle significant problems ranging from substance misuse and anti-social behaviour through to mental health problems and persistent absence from school.

By widening thinking or 'thinking family' (Gopfert and others 2004), it is possible to better understand individual members in terms of the pressures on them; the role they play; and the knock-on effects of their feelings or behaviour on others, and vice versa.

It can be helpful to explore with individual service users (or all family members) what a typical day is like for them. By thinking about what happens for one person in this kind of detail, it can make it easier to imagine how others who live with them experience this. Gaining a clearer understanding of these factors will enable services to better support families, identify where gaps and needs are and target helpful interventions.

At the service level, participants in the Building Resilience project reported a variety of ways in which their services were moving towards meeting family needs better. One agency was using grants to fund family day trips and outings; others were developing family rooms within psychiatric facilities; and another was developing a 'family visiting coordinator' post to assist with maintaining contact where parents were hospitalised or in treatment. Some services had parental mental health interest groups or networks; and another was working with local schools to increase their awareness of the needs of children of substance-misusing parents.

Practice example 4 shows a parental mental health service operating a 'whole family' approach.

Practice example 4: Family Action's Building Bridges project

Family Action's Building Bridges service has been around since 1999. It is a model aimed at supporting families with a range of multiple complex needs including where parents have severe and enduring mental health problems. For example where the model is commissioned by Tower Hamlets Primary Care Trust the focus is on intervening early so as to reduce the risk of escalation of an adult's mental health problems, and thus the need for acute hospitalisation of adults and of care orders for children, and to improve safeguarding and development outcomes for children. It is usually delivered in families' homes and seeks to meet the needs of each family member by supporting the role of the adult as parent or carer and responding to the separate, related needs of the child. Overall Building Bridges is currently delivered in Edenbridge, Lewisham, Hackney, Southwark, Luton, Newham, Tower Hamlets, Coventry and Greenwich.

The service was inspired by research showing that, while there is a need for social workers to consider the risk of significant harm to the child resulting from a parent's mental health, not all severe parental mental health problems result in harm to the child, particularly where the adult is supported to gain insight into their mental health problems, to parent positively, and to prioritise family tasks ('Parents with Psychiatric Problems' by Diana Cassell and Rosalyn Coleman in *Assessment of Parental Psychiatric and Psychological Contributions*, eds. Reder and Lucey, Blackwell Synergy, 1995). These latter activities are core to the delivery of the Building Bridges service.

Building Bridge's *Think Family* approach to parents with mental health problems has been reinforced by more recent national policy initiatives and research, for example, the Social Exclusion Unit's 2007 *'Reaching Out: Think Family'* review on Families at Risk that examined the challenges in engaging with and supporting families with multiple complex needs.

The practice criteria and arrangements for referrals to the service depend on local commissioning. However, around a third of referrals come from children's services, followed closely by adult mental services, self-referrals and voluntary organisations.

The starting point for the service is families' perceptions of their needs and their goals. It is delivered by professional Family Support Workers who provide practical as well as emotional support and who are available at times when others services are not, e.g. bedtimes, weekends and bank holidays.

Activities can include:

- engaging children in the family in an understanding of their parent's mental health problems
- helping a parent manage a child's challenging behaviour accompanying parents and their children to Sure Start/other services groups so they gain the confidence to use these services regularly.
- practical steps towards addressing poverty, i.e. signposting to benefits checks or
- securing grants to obtaining essential household items that are missing.

Impact measures

In 2004, Family Action decided to adopt formal evaluation tools across the Building Bridges projects that would enable the organisation, and the individual projects, to measure the impact of the service provided to parents and children. The impact of the service on the family is measured through the Index of Family Relationships (parents); the Kansas Parental Satisfaction Scale (parents); Rosenberg Self Esteem Scale (children 11 and over), and the depression rating scale (children under 11). The impact on the wider community has been assessed through the number of children on the local child protection register and the number of adults on the care programme approach.

Overall outcomes of Building Bridges from a recent independent evaluation (2011):
Over two cohorts of families with a range of multiple complex needs from 2004 to 2010 Building Bridges reduced the need for the following:

- Care Programme Approach by 47 per cent
- the child protection register by 54 per cent
- local authority care by 70 per cent
- the Common Assessment Framework Team Around the Child Single Agency by 52 per cent
- the Common Assessment Team Around the Child Multi-Agency by 67 per cent
- and for Children In Need by 54 per cent.

For further information contact Jayne Stokes jayne.stokes@family-action.org.uk or visit www.family-action.org.uk to read the full Building Bridges evaluation.

A whole-family approach includes proactive efforts by service providers to engage fathers as well as mothers. In particular, fathers who live separately from their children but still have contact with them are an important part of children's lives, and they need to be considered and engaged more by professionals. Families welcome services that are inclusive of fathers in their approach (Kroll and Taylor 2003). For further discussion of the need for services to be better geared up to include fathers, see page 92.

There also needs to be more attention paid to both the needs of extended family members and the potential contribution to assessments and support that they can make. When relatives are significantly involved in supporting families, professionals should avoid making assumptions that they are 'coping' (Hart and Powell 2006). It can be particularly difficult for wider family members to bring up their own support needs, which can arise from the practicalities of providing support, the emotional toll of worrying about their family members, divided loyalties, guilt and conflicts. Relatives may also need support and information to help them understand mental health needs or substance issues.

Similarly, kinship carers often experience conflicting loyalties, anger and worry about the parents, and guilt about their own role and responsibility in the parent's problems. The wider needs of kinship carers, and agencies' responses to their needs are discussed elsewhere.

The following sections explore some of the particular kinds of support that children and parents tend to value, although many of the features of supportive services for parents will also apply to extended family members and kinship carers too.

Support to parents

Research and literature consistently shows that, when asked what they want, the majority of parents with mental health problems referred first to what they wanted for their children: 'to feel ordinary and to get early attention and support if their life is disrupted' (Tunnard 2004). When asked about what would help them in terms of support, there is much overlap between what those affected by parental substance misuse and mental health issues have said, although some differences will occur within and between the needs and responses of these two groups. Parents often report feeling undermined. They do not want to be judged or in fear of their children being removed if they ask for help. They require professionals to be proactive in giving reassurance about negative perceptions they think they may hold about them, as they are used to stigmatising and discriminating attitudes (Tunnard 2004). While this section uses the term 'parent' throughout, much will apply to alternative carers or other affected family members.

Help in their own right

Many parents, particularly with mental health problems, say they want help to meet their parental responsibilities. Parents whose children undertake caring roles generally want support to relieve the burden on the child (a few parents with severe mental health problems were not troubled by children caring for them, but most didn't want to be so reliant on their children) (Tunnard 2004).

Practice example 5 shows a holistic service for families affected by parental substance misuse which gives support to help parents and children play together.

Practice example 5: CAN – Northamptonshire

CAN offers a holistic service to families where parents recognise that their substance use is impacting on the care of their children. As well as undertaking individual counselling, groupwork, and advice and support with adults, CAN Children's Workers work on a one-to-one basis with children aged 5 to 12 of service users. The Children's Workers use lots of tactile resources to help with the communication of feelings through play. This includes the use of sand trays, puppets, board games, books, dolls and figures, paints, play dough etc.

The parent(s)/carer(s) are involved in the work with the children from the start. They are invited to attend an appointment in order that the Children's Worker can complete an assessment for the child/ren. They are then invited to attend review sessions with the worker every six weeks to discuss the work that has been completed with the child/ren and to help them communicate in an adult way with their child about their substance use issues and its impact on the child.

It was partly during these sessions that it was identified that some service users find it difficult to play with their children. This could be for a variety of reasons. It might be that the client did not experience play with their own parent(s) or that their misuse is their primary concern and play is not high on the agenda. In response to this need, CAN staff organise 'Play Workshops' throughout the year and with individual families working with the service, which have proved very successful. Clients with children are invited to come

---

along and do various activities together. The team are on hand to join in as well as answer any questions the parent(s)/carer(s) might have.

For further information about CAN, contact:
Ellie Davies and Sue Becker at CAN Northampton 01604 627027
Anthea Spence (Children's Worker) 01933 271879 or 01604 627027

CAN Young Peoples Team – Service

CAN Young Peoples Team is a free, confidential drug and alcohol service for young people under the age of 19 and their families/carers in Northamptonshire. CAN YP Team aim to provide information, education, advice and treatment to young people in relation to drug and alcohol use.

Who can access CAN YP team?

- a young person who is concerned about someone else's drug use including parents, carers, siblings or friends.
- a young person who is using but would like to reduce the harm caused.
- a young person who would like to reduce their drug use or stop.
- a young person who needs an opiate substitute prescription (methadone, subutex).
- a young person who needs support into inpatient detox for alcohol dependency.

What is on offer?

- Confidential information, education and harm reduction advice around drug and alcohol use.
- Referral into treatment.
- BBV screening.
- Family work.
- Relapse work and Aftercare.
- Group information, education and harm reduction sessions for targeted groups.

Work with Looked after Children.

- Dedicated Schools Liaison worker.
- Exploitation prevention and awareness work.
- Joint work with Youth Offending Service and the Police.
- Advice for professionals.
- Professionals training sessions.

Contact details:
Admin base at
76 St Giles Street
Northampton NN1 1JW. Tel: 08450 556246
email: ypadmin@can.org.uk
Fax: 01604 930035

Practical and emotional support

Whilst some parents want parenting advice, research by the ESRC Families and Social Capital Research Group at South Bank University (Edwards and Gillies 2005) shows that most would prefer concrete, practical services. Services that 'lighten the load' or alleviate stress, such as help with transporting children to school, are valued (Tunnard 2004). Also, parents appreciate being able to gain support from other parents and being enabled to have a break. Substance-misusing parents particularly value access to informal support during difficult times, and help with practical and emotional problems that might not be substance related (Kroll and Taylor 2003).

Emotional support that parents indicate would be helpful includes:

- help in coping with children's needs when they have emotional and behavioural difficulties
- support to help family members understand each other
- counselling or someone to talk to informally, or both
- assistance in finding alternative coping styles, if they are needing to change, or to reduce the use of their usual strategies.

Preventative support and help in promoting resilience

Professional involvement at an early stage is wanted by many parents and not just during a crisis. Heide Lloyd (Falkov 1998) draws on her own experience of parenting with mental health problems and suggests that parents can benefit from doing things to help reduce stress, for example by having enough food in to cover meals for at least two days in case they become tired or unwell, having a few convenience meals to hand, preparing lunch boxes and clothes for the children for the next day in advance. Such strategies, if individually developed and tailored, can help people to feel in control and 'stop the day seeming so overwhelming'.

Childcare support to be available when needed and services which help to reduce isolation are also wanted; and there is a greater need for follow-up and aftercare services than is generally currently available.

Practice example 6: Family Action case study from Building Bridges project

As outlined in practice example 4 Building Bridges is a professional, intensive, home-based family support service designed to respond to families with multiple complex needs. This is a case study from one of the London projects.

Case study

Mrs A, the mother of a two-year-old girl, was referred to Family Action's Building Bridges service in London. She had already been admitted to hospital for her psychotic condition once. She had become overweight, anxious and mainly housebound relying on her husband to care for her and her daughter. Neither of the couple was working and they were in debt. At times when Mrs A improved, Mr A then seemed to sabotage her progress. One serious incident involved Mr A filming Mrs A's psychotic episode and pushing child A to Mrs A when the child was very obviously distressed and crying. Their daughter was beginning to display language development and behavioural problems, which were increasing unhelpful stress on Mrs A.

Approach

The Building Bridges service worked with Mrs A and her husband and daughter to understand the whole family's needs. The key support worker helped Mrs A to develop an insight into her mental health condition and to establish a routine based on earlier waking and bedtimes, healthier eating and more exercise, all of which are known to support compliance with medication and impact positively on mental health in their own right. The worker accompanied Mrs A on shopping trips and to a local leisure centre to give her confidence in leaving the house. She showed Mrs A the importance of engaging with her daughter, and how she could play with her in more creative ways. She demonstrated to Mr and Mrs A how their inconsistent parenting approaches to their daughter were causing some of her behavioural problems; and engaged Mr A in understanding how he could at times seem to undermine Mrs A as a parent. Mr and Mrs A were helped to understand the impact of this on the child.

Outcomes

Since Family Action intervened Mrs A and her daughter are exhibiting much improved parent–child attachment. Her daughter's speech, behaviour and self-esteem have improved considerably. She has been found a nursery place close to home. All in all, she has been put on a firmer footing for succeeding at primary school. Mrs A obtained a job but the stress involved in the change seemed to threaten to precipitate a relapse. She wants to try again in the future. In the meantime she is studying childcare and volunteering for a mental health charity locally, has made some friends at the leisure centre with whom she is going swimming regularly, and has lost more than a stone in weight. Mr A is taking driving lessons and volunteering in a community centre and has stopped smoking. The couple have reviewed their household budget to reduce their debt; and have obtained permanent housing in better quality condition.

Learning points

- To secure improvements in outcomes for the child, the needs of the whole family should be approached holistically.
- As is shown by much research into what works in family support, the role of a key worker who works consistently in partnership with the family is crucial.
- An all-important foundation for securing the improvement in the child's outcomes is the creation of routines and structures to assist the parent with managing their difficulties. In respect of mental health this can include support with compliance with medication, developing a programme of regular sleep and exercise, and creating a healthy diet.
- Other adults in the household may not have a mental health problem, but their behaviours may be impacting negatively on the parent–child relationships, and the child's behaviour and development. They may need support to understand why.
- Support needs to be given to parents not only with their relationships within the home but also with wider communities, for example with using local services and accessing volunteering and training opportunities. Once this is given parents can begin to generate their own social networks.
- To secure positive economic outcomes for the child support may also be required for practical issues such as housing and debt reduction.

For further information contact Jayne Stokes jayne.stokes@family-action.org.uk or visit www.family-action.org.uk to read the full Building Bridges evaluation.

Flexible and holistic support services

Support services that are flexible and responsive to individual need, do not impose expectations, and recognise the environmental factors that affect people, are valued. Those that make proactive efforts to ensure provision is acceptable and inclusive of fathers are better able to engage and support them. For all parents, the opportunity to choose from a range of support services promotes their usefulness and uptake.

Voluntary services can often be tailored to family circumstances and play a very important role in supporting parents.

If parents can get their needs and those of the child met in the same place, the child is more likely to be seen and their needs addressed. Also, if parents can get a range of issues addressed in one place they are more likely to attend the service. 'One stop shops' have been mentioned many times as a useful means of service provision.

Utilising services can be time-consuming and potentially stressful, particularly if childcare needs or other access issues are not addressed by the service. Services that are able to offer flexible appointment times, a choice of home visits or office/centre visits, and drop-in facilities are more likely to be utilised.

Drawing specialists into convenient or comfortable (for service users) settings, such as trusted local voluntary or community services, can minimise the stress and anxiety that can come with having lots of appointments with different people and in different places.

Some specific service deficits, cited in surveys and studies as requiring improvements in order to better meet parents' support needs, include better family-friendly facilities in psychiatric hospitals; mother and baby units for women experiencing postnatal psychosis; and support with bonding when babies in special care units have withdrawal symptoms (Morris and Wates 2006).

Information

Parents would like to be given accessible information regarding the context of statutory services' role when they are involved with them, such as information about procedures, confidentiality and professionals' powers (Tunnard 2004).

Information about medication and its effects and, for substance-misusing parents, information – sensitively provided – about the impact of parents' substance use on their children is also wanted (Morris and Wates 2006).

Direct support to children

When asked what has helped them, children tend to refer to help from family members, informal mentors and friends rather than the actions of paid professionals. Although most children prefer to talk to peers of their own age, knowing there is an adult with a listening ear at the right time can prove crucial.

An awareness of the potential helpfulness of sources of informal support is vital if professionals are to ensure that their intervention does not weaken these links.

Considering how support can strengthen and build on resilience factors for children (outlined in Chapter 3) is an important starting point when considering appropriate support for children.

Many children compartmentalise aspects of their lives in order to cope with their situation, and many experience feelings of guilt and a sense of responsibility for their parents' problems. They need help, encouragement and sometimes skilled intervention to enable them to share their feelings.

When asked about their experiences of stress, whereas adults tend to point to major stressful life events, children and young people refer to 'daily hassles' (Newman and Blackburn 2002) such as falling out with friends. Such events and stresses should not be overlooked given their capacity to cause feelings of stress in children, because cumulative or chronic stress presents potentially long-term risks to children and young people.

In her review of the research and literature relating to parental mental ill health, Tunnard (2004) listed the following responses of children as to what they wanted in terms of support.

They wanted:

- above all for their parent or parents to be well
- for themselves to be cared for
- to get the attention they need
- for their parents to be able to meet other parents in similar circumstances
- information – children and young people want to understand:
    - the reason for their parent's mood swings
    - medication
    - the causes of mental illness
    - symptoms
    - likely consequences of health problems
    - how to deal with problems
    - when to call a GP
    - how to notice changes in mood and their significance
- help in coping with embarrassing or bizarre behaviours that their parent exhibits in public, in school, or in front of their peers
- information to be age-appropriate and not overloading
- someone to talk to
- opportunities to relax and have fun.

According to Tunnard (2002a), children affected by parental substance misuse have many similar wishes and often need:

- time away
- reassurance that their parent's drug use is not their fault or responsibility
- help with losses and separations
- help and reassurance concerning fears of being removed from their home or parent (real or imagined)
- opportunities for group discussion and activities (these may be inclusive as opposed to specialist, as this is often better received and has benefits)
- the above to be in tandem with changes at home (perhaps brought about by a parent benefiting from treatment)
- either individual or family work to help the child to find ways of coping with changes, new rules and boundaries
- respite and recreation opportunities.

Practice example 7 shows how coordinated support to both a mother and her child can enhance their relationship and improve their circumstances. It illustrates family-focused direct work in action.

Practice example 7: ADAS UK

Synopsis of family situation

At the time of referral to the Child Therapy service at ADAS, Jack* was 8. His mother, Sarah*, contacted ADAS as she had concerns about his behaviour, describing him as withdrawing from her and trying to self-harm. Sarah had a history of drug use and alcohol misuse, although at the time of referral, she was no longer using drugs but was still binge-drinking. Jack's father, Dean, also had a history of drug use and, at the time of referral, was reported to be still using. Sarah and Dean no longer lived together and there was a history of domestic violence between Sarah and Dean. Sarah and Jack had recently spent time in a refuge and Jack had intermittent contact with his father.

An initial referral meeting was set up by the child therapist with Sarah. The aim of this meeting was to explore with Sarah what her concerns were regarding her son and also to obtain a fuller history of the family's main experiences. During this first meeting, Sarah talked about her long history of physical and mental ill health, her substance misuse difficulties, and her recognition of the impact all this had had on Jack, both when he was a baby and in recent years. Sarah admitted that Jack had taken on a great deal of responsibility, especially in looking after her. Sarah explained that Jack frequently missed school when she was too ill to leave the home and would take on household tasks such as cleaning and preparing simple meals for both of them. Sarah explained that for a while, she had had a support worker from the refuge that she and Jack lived in but since being rehoused, that support had ceased. Sarah and Jack were fairly isolated as a family unit in the new community they were living in. Following years of chaotic family life, Sarah had become estranged from most of her family and Jack had little contact with his father's family. Although Sarah was no longer using drugs, she was finding it increasingly difficult to cope with daily life stressors and was concerned about the risk of starting to use again. She was also worried about her binge-drinking as she felt her alcohol intake was increasing.

During this first meeting and in a second follow-up meeting, the child therapist discussed the option of individual counselling for Sarah, some relapse prevention sessions and the possibility of Sarah working with a family support worker at ADAS. The child therapist also discussed what protective factors, if any, were in place when Sarah and Jack were alone at home. The child therapist also talked to Sarah about undertaking a CAF (Common Assessment Framework) with her and Jack as it was deemed that Jack was a 'child in need'. Sarah said that Jack's school had already completed something similar and the child therapist sought consent from Sarah to contact Jack's school and find out if anything was already in place. Sarah agreed to these suggestions. It was also agreed that Sarah would start her own counselling before play therapy commenced with Jack so as to ensure that Sarah was able to emotionally contain Jack and to support him through his therapeutic intervention. The child therapist agreed to meet with Sarah on a regular basis so as to help her think of ways to facilitate communication between Sarah and Jack.

Action

Counselling for Sarah started shortly after the initial meetings with the Child Therapy service, and Jack's own play therapy sessions started a few weeks after that. In addition to that support, following an assessment by a support worker at ADAS, Sarah was found to be alcohol dependent and was referred to the local Community Drug and Alcohol Team (CDAT) where she was prescribed antabuse to help her reduce her alcohol intake.

When a family is seen at ADAS by both the Adult and Child and Family services, regular family meetings are held which are attended by the counsellor/s, child therapist and family support workers who are involved with the adult/s and child/ren. Confidentiality is maintained for both the adult/s and child/ren during these meetings but any issues that seem to be presenting difficulties for the family as a unit are discussed and any child protection concerns are highlighted and duly addressed; practical issues are also raised such as housing or financial issues. If these are seen to be causing further stress for the parent and/or child, the ADAS support worker is asked to work with the family. Communication between mother and son was raised by both the adult counsellor and the child therapist as being a difficulty and this was addressed with Sarah and Jack in a variety of ways. The Child Therapy service offers regular review meetings to parents in which themes and issues arising from the child's sessions are discussed. These were held with Sarah but in addition, she was also offered the opportunity to attend parenting support meetings with the family worker at ADAS where parenting strategies were discussed. Sarah attended these meetings regularly.

During the course of Sarah and Jack's engagement with ADAS, substantial progress was made by both mother and child. By having a safe space in which to express and explore his thoughts and feelings through the medium of play, Jack was able to move from being a withdrawn, highly anxious child to one whose self-esteem developed and who became able to express himself verbally. His relationship with his mother improved as Sarah's own self-esteem and confidence grew. Sarah did not revert back to using drugs and was able to address her drinking difficulties through her counselling and the support from CDAT. The family worker was instrumental in helping Sarah regain her role as mother and this then allowed Jack to give up his 'parent' role that he had adopted. Sarah also learnt to listen to her son and to spend positive time with him. Although attempts were made by the Child and Family service at ADAS to engage with Jack's father, these were never successful and Jack's relationship with Dean continued to be difficult for him. Sarah was supported in trying to establish consistent contact between Jack and Dean but by the time this family left ADAS after just over a year of attending, contact between father and son continued to be problematic.

The relative success of the above intervention with Sarah and Jack was due to close collaboration between the Adult and Child and Family services at ADAS but also between ADAS and statutory services such as CDAT, as well as the child's school. Information was shared amongst the professionals working with the family and the mother, and where appropriate, with the child too. This enabled the mother to access the support she so badly needed which, in turn, helped to ameliorate the home situation, thus making it a healthier environment, physically and emotionally, for both mother and son to live in.

*The names in the above example are fictitious and some details have been changed to protect the identity of the family involved.

Contact details:

Philomena Lawrence, Chief Executive, ADAS
phil@adasuk.org
Elise Refalo, Children's Support Therapist, Children's Support Service, ADAS
elise@adasuk.org admin@adasuk.org

In direct work, going at a pace appropriate to children's needs and circumstances is not an easy balance to strike and requires skill and awareness of the child's communication needs and level of development.

Participants on the Building Resilience project that provided direct work to children varied in their views about timing, with some not starting therapeutic work until there was a reasonable degree of stability in the child's life and others offering therapeutic work while things were chaotic as the child's needs were so high at that time. They all considered, before embarking on the work, whether there was a significant adult who could support and contain the child while they were receiving counselling or therapeutic work. Sometimes work with parents was undertaken first to better prepare them to support the child (see Practice example 2). In some cases, this turned out to be all that was needed and the child's problems resolved without their own therapeutic work commencing.

As with adults, identifying children's goals, strengths, likes and dislikes provides a useful foundation for working with them. Engaging them in activities they enjoy often results in them communicating a lot more freely than when using more formal approaches.

Some participants on the Building Resilience project used trigger cards, manuals, workbooks, sand play and games in their direct work with children and found these approaches effective. Communicating by email and text has also increased the likelihood of children and young people keeping in touch with services.

Practice example 8 concerns a service with a focus on early intervention. In this instance a project for Asian teenage girls has enhanced accessibility to service users and engaged their parents, community leaders and other professionals.

Practice example 8: Newham Asian Women's Project

Zindaagi (meaning 'life') is a project led by Newham Asian Women's Project (NAWP). The project delivers a range of services aimed at reducing the incidents of self-harm and suicide amongst South Asian women and girls; and actively works to promote their emotional well-being and self-empowerment.

Our early intervention project involves workshops and drop-in sessions in schools as well as after school clubs – **Teens@NAWP** and **Girls Allowed** for young women. Workshops are delivered on a range of issues, such as confidence building, self-esteem, stress management etc. To increase accessibility, we have adapted the way we work and after sessions drop the girls back home. Parents feel more comfortable seeing the children being dropped off, knowing who they are with. As a result, we have built a trusting relationship with parents who then allow their daughters to go on residential weekend trips with the group as well.

Providing workshops and our service in schools has proved to be very successful, especially given that many South Asian parents do not want their children to be out after school. Having a presence in school provides them with the opportunity to access services they may not otherwise be able to, as well as ensures that it is a setting they are comfortable in.

In order to communicate more effectively with young women, we have also begun to use an office mobile phone. This allows our young women to text us or give us a missed call if they need to talk. This is a medium of communication they are comfortable using. We are also able to then text them with reminders of meetings etc. This is a method that is age appropriate and we believe has enabled larger numbers of young women to access our services.

Our services are user led and developed. We consistently consult with service users on their needs and how they would like the service to develop. Creative methods of evaluation have involved getting the young women to keep a diary of how they felt before and after activities, what's worked for them and what hasn't and also allows us to gauge their emotional growth.

In addition, to increase professionals' awareness of the cultural issues impacting young women and the effect these may have on the way they engage with mental health services, we deliver training to professionals highlighting some of these cultural concepts.

We also work within the community with faith leaders who we find are often the first point of contact for many BAMER young women experiencing emotional distress. Providing them with the knowledge and information to appropriately support their clients is important and also allows us to dispel some of the myths that are held by the community at large about mental health.

Quotes

I used to get bullied and the bullying workshop has helped me learn how to deal with bullies ... I feel happier that now I know I can do something about it ... I feel that I would be able to talk to Teens [youth group] or to my parents if it happens again.

(young Asian woman)

I felt it was a very safe and warm environment that generated in-depth discussions. The trainers were knowledgeable and made us very comfortable from the start. Raised my awareness of self-harm and issues of the Asian communities.

(professional's evaluation of self-harm training, and young Asian women)

For further information about the project, contact:

Zindaagi Team
Newham Asian Women's Project
661 Barking Road, Plaistow
London E13 9EX
Tel: 0208 472 0528, 079 6164 4088
E: info@nawp.org

6. How can services support families more effectively at the strategic level?

This chapter examines the provision of effective support services for children and families at the strategic level of service development and planning. It discusses: information collection and needs analysis; funding; joint commissioning and joint planning; joint working culture and joint working protocols; crossover posts; user involvement; training and skills development; evaluation; coherent policies; dual diagnosis; kinship care; raising awareness and challenging stigma; promoting more accessible services for black and minority ethnic communities; and increasing the capacity to involve fathers.

Information collection and needs analysis

The first step towards improving services and increasing coordination of services, and in making a credible case for increased funding, is reaching a clearer understanding of the numbers and needs of families affected nationally and locally by parental mental health problems and substance misuse issues. The first stage of this process is to understand local needs, and this is underpinned by the local Joint Strategic Needs Assessment (JSNA). The coalition government is implementing wide-ranging changes to the commissioning and delivery of NHS, public health and social care provision. A key aim of this is to achieve better integration of health and social care services. To aid partnership working at local level it is envisaged that the Health and Wellbeing Board in every local authority area will be responsible for preparing the JSNA and the joint Health and Well-being Strategy. The Health and Well-being Board will bring together the Directors of Adult and Children's Services and the Director of Public Health, providing a forum through which decisions may be taken on the needs of vulnerable families.

Much information is already available but not being pulled together; and other data is unavailable because it is not broken down sufficiently to highlight specific areas of need. Local authorities themselves (children and adults' services, youth services, benefits, leisure, housing) hold much information that could already be utilised. Primary Care and NHS Trusts, primary care practices, schools, district councils, police, Youth Offending Teams, Connexions services/their equivalent and local voluntary community and private sectors all hold significant amounts of information about their users' presenting needs. Other data may come from anonymised Common Assessment Forms, complaints systems, central government (including Office for National Statistics) and inspectorates as well as from other national private and voluntary organisations.

The now archived DfES/DH guidance, *Joint Planning and Commissioning Framework for Children, Young People and Maternity services* (2006), states that the information collected should be able to be broken down by variables such as ethnicity, gender, sexual orientation, religion, learning disability, looked after status, risk of criminality, geographical location and access to services. If such information can also be broken down to show the main areas of difficulty or need encountered by users, including where there are parental mental ill health or substance misuse issues, domestic violence, physical disabilities, and where there are dual or multiple issues, this will be a vital step in increasing the understanding and capacity to prioritise and target services more appropriately.

Adequate funding

Time and again participants on the Building Resilience project raised the difficulties they had in providing the services that they knew were required by service users due to limitations in their funding. Many of the smaller specialist teams – such as substance misuse, mother and baby, or alcohol services – received funding on a short-term basis only, so much of their time and energy went into trying to secure more. This affects the way in which services are able to develop and the focus of their skills and efforts. Many had waiting lists or had to raise their eligibility thresholds in order to gate-keep their resources. So, whilst most are aware of the importance of early intervention and preventative work, it is often not possible in practice for many agencies to undertake this. Typical threshold criteria might, for example, be that there is a risk of self-harm, child protection issues, domestic violence or someone coming out of detoxification. Volunteers and students were utilised in some services as a way of bolstering their service capacity.

Whilst there are no easy solutions, it is worth considering what more, if anything, can be done within existing resources to either influence this and bring about more funding opportunities or to better target the funds that are available.

Firstly, in order to make a case for more resources it is essential that more be done to identify gaps in services, unmet needs and the consequences of them continuing to go unmet, as discussed above. Secondly, pooling the resources of different agencies, so that they can be channelled into services which meet cross-cutting needs, can be more efficient and meet needs more effectively than single services providing for supposedly different aspects of individual or family needs. It is important that service providers work cooperatively to maximise their resources. The alternative is not only increased fragmentation of services, but also different agencies competing for funding or contracts for the same issue.

Joint commissioning and joint planning

Joint commissioning, for example between children's services and primary care trusts (or their replacements, GP-led Clinical Commissioning groups), is a very important step that should be considered where possible.

The Children Act 2004 provides an overview for an increasing focus on joint planning and commissioning. The DfES/DH *Joint Planning and Commissioning Framework for Children, Young People and Maternity Services* (2006) guidance set out a framework for children's trusts, for use in planning and commissioning, in order to promote best outcomes for children and young people. The National Service Framework for Mental Health similarly identifies a need for more joint commissioning and greater service integration.

Whilst a full move towards jointly planned and commissioned services is going to take time, there is much that can be achieved on an individual service or service area level, and it is better to start small than not at all. It is worth planners and partners considering how they can build on existing services and arrangements in the shorter term. Multi-agency approaches and bringing resources together, for example in crossover posts (discussed below) – where a worker from one service, such as adult mental health, is co-located within another, such as a children and families' team – can make a positive impact on providing a more integrated response to service users' needs.

Joint working culture

In the Building Resilience workshops, participants were asked about the factors they saw as supporting joint working. Co-location of a variety of professionals meant services were better placed to meet users' holistic needs and tended to be seen as the best and easiest model from which to provide effective services. They also highlighted the importance of a culture of joint working being embedded throughout the organisation at all levels, with a clear commitment centred around service users' needs that is clearly led by senior managers. The Commission for Social Care Inspection (2006) also highlighted the importance of a clear and explicit vision of parent support being communicated throughout adults' and children's organisations as a starting point in improving services.

The need for good communication in its many and varied forms was, not surprisingly, raised most often by participants in the workshops. Examples such as key workers from relevant but different services meeting face to face regularly, as a matter of course, were seen as crucial. Such mechanisms create opportunities for reducing repetition of assessment for service users; and allowing for better preparation, follow-up and clarity of understanding of individual users' needs. Regular direct contact between professionals in different services was also a feature of some of the services that appeared to be successful in establishing a whole-family approach. Such meetings were useful in strengthening relationships; awareness; and systems such as referral processes, joint visits, assessments and care plans.

Formal meetings, or for example attendance at referral meetings of other services, were seen as only part of the picture. 'Getting about' – by which participants meant physically being in the same place, getting practitioners' faces, names and roles known across services – was seen as vital. Where staff know at least one person in a related service whom they feel able to access, collaboration is far more likely to occur and, most crucially, to occur at an earlier stage of intervention. Also, if workers are enabled and indeed expected to share their skills and knowledge and access each other's expertise – and supported in doing so by clear guidance and protocols as discussed below – this will improve their ability to respond holistically, confidently and appropriately to users' needs. Being able to simply 'have a chat' across service boundaries, even when thresholds for the other service are not met, is an essential part of preventative working and is supported by cultivating relationships with individuals. A high turnover of staff in some services makes this more of a challenge, as do the demands on individual workers' time. Hence the importance of clear direction from senior staff about these issues, factoring in networking and advice-giving into the workloads of staff and teams.

The Social Care Institute for Excellence (SCIE) has developed a range of resources on parental mental health and child welfare (including dual diagnosis), and provides good practice examples. (See http://www.scie.org.uk/topic/people/peoplewithmentalhealthproblems/familieschildrenwhohavementalhealthproblems

Joint working protocols

Well-implemented joint working protocols – guidelines that set out the way in which two or more services should respond to given situations – are not a substitute for skilled practice, but are a useful starting point in providing a foundation for working practices and clarity of expectations. They should provide clear instructions and requirements and be easy to use. However, in a 1998 study carried out by the National Institute for Social Work (NISW), it was found that less than half of the responding agencies had developed working protocols in relation to families affected by parental mental health or substance misuse.

The Social Care Institute for Excellence (SCIE, formerly NISW), in its 2003 report *Families That Have Alcohol and Mental Health Problems: A template for partnership working* (Kearney and others), provides suggestions regarding protocol development and implementation. It stresses the need for protocols to arise from a collaboration between the relevant agencies as this is a useful and necessary exercise in itself. Protocols should:

> be the result of agencies working together to produce it while reaching a common understanding of roles, values and actions

The process involved should:

> reinforce and set out the steps to be taken in order to work together in joint assessment, care planning, management of risk, monitoring and reviewing in individual cases

(p.4)

Protocols, if they are to be useful in practice, should be founded on an understanding of the needs they are hoping to meet and the outcomes to be achieved. These should be identified at the outset, alongside a consideration of who to involve from relevant agencies and service users in drawing up the protocols. There will need to be a clear understanding and statement within the protocol of the relevant legislation and policy guidance within which the particular agencies are working. It will be necessary to consider what's in place already – such as agreed referral routes or forms, what's working and where there are gaps in arrangements.

The guidance goes on to highlight the need to reach a consensus on the values and principles underpinning the working arrangements; the vocabulary used; and to explicitly define some key concepts, such as:

- confidentiality
- treatability
- young carers
- the boundaries of responsibility
- the standards that the protocols aim to uphold.

The development of protocols can be very time-consuming and to ensure that they are 'owned' across the organisations requires all stakeholders to be fully involved in devising them. This ownership is essential to its effective implementation. One way of underlining ownership is for senior staff from the relevant organisations to sign the final document and a joint introductory statement, hence making it clear to their respective staff that the guidance applies to them.

To reduce the time spent in producing protocols, agencies can refer to the many useful ones already in existence and adapt them accordingly (see Further resources and the SCIE website). More overarching protocols, such as child protection procedures, can be used as a basis; to which can be added supplementary sections, for example to cover issues of parental mental health problems or substance misuse. However, it is important that this does not mean that some of the essential groundwork described above, in collaborating with stakeholders, is by-passed in order to save time.

It is not uncommon for agencies to have protocols that have not been implemented effectively, either because the groundwork wasn't done, so they are not workable, or because in reality they become no more than paper documents on shelves. To ensure that protocols are implemented and disseminated effectively, it helps to ensure that they are widely accessible, backed up by launches and training, referred to regularly in supervision and practice development activities, and included as an essential part of new workers' induction programmes. They also need to be regularly updated and their outcomes evaluated.

Within the Building Resilience workshops, participants told us that a lack of understanding of each other's roles and the legislative basis for working contributed to the difficulties they encountered in working confidently across professional boundaries, along with unclear referral pathways and information-sharing arrangements.

The most important factors in improving interagency practice were the clear articulation of services' responsibilities and of mechanisms for challenging when these responsibilities do not appear to be met. Many saw joint working protocols as an important part of bringing such clarity and reducing misunderstanding between agencies about what sort of response could be expected of them in particular circumstances. They stressed the need for regular feedback; and for mechanisms whereby relevant users and professionals could review how the protocols were working in practice. In addition, they wanted the training of all affected agencies to include clear and regular reference to the protocols, so that the guidance remained 'live' and relevant.

Coherent policies on specific issues: Dual diagnosis and kinship care

Dual diagnosis

This is an area in which coherent policies and guidance, within and between agencies, could improve the experience and outcomes for users and families. Without clear guidance there is often a tension between services which are each primarily set up to deal with one issue or 'service user type'. For example, when mental ill health and substance misuse occur together, practitioners told us of the pressure they encounter to 'narrow their vision' to the focus that is considered to be within their agency remit, and therefore 'separate issues falsely'. Similarly, in certain circumstances, in order to ensure service users are viewed as meeting threshold criteria, there can be an increased emphasis on trying to find information to support the fact that a service user 'fits a label' so they can access the service.

Participants on the Building Resilience project talked of the disputes that often take place between services as to where the responsibility to the service user lies and how the work should proceed. For example, some hold the view that a person's substance use needs to be addressed before their mental health problems can be treated effectively; but for others it's vice versa. It is more useful to work towards a model where mental health services are able to access or include support for those with drug or alcohol misuse problems; and vice versa. There are also differences in opinion within different services regarding confidentiality and where the boundaries lie. In short, dual diagnosis seems to be responded to at a service level with dual stigma, increased bureaucracy, delays and less efficiency.

Clear guidance and policies regarding dual diagnosis are seen as helpful in addressing this; and national guidance on dual diagnosis does exist. The Department of Health's *Mental Health Policy Implementation Guide: Dual diagnosis good practice guide* (2002) is clear in its guidance that mental health services should take a coordinating role:

> *Individuals with these dual problems deserve high quality, patient-focused and integrated care.* **This should be delivered within mental health services** *[their emphasis]. This policy is referred to as 'mainstreaming'. Patients should not be shunted between different sets of services or put at risk of dropping out of care completely. 'Mainstreaming' will not reduce the role of drug and alcohol services, which will continue to treat the majority of people with substance misuse problems and to advise on substance misuse issues.*

The Department of Health further stresses the need for definitions to be agreed between agencies and for all relevant staff to be trained and equipped to work with dual diagnosis. They suggest that specialist teams of dual diagnosis workers be formed, as a useful lever of support for mainstream mental health services; and Building Resilience project participants also reported the helpfulness of dual diagnosis worker posts, where these existed.

There is also a need for clear arrangements to be agreed for when support with mental health is needed but where problems are not defined as severe and enduring. This links back to the need for joint working protocols, discussed earlier.

Kinship care

Many children in need of substitute care, either temporarily or permanently, are placed with members of their extended family or friends. These kinship or family and friends carers, as they are also known, play a significant role in families affected by parental mental health or substance misuse difficulties. Where workable, these can be the most positive option for children and families and most local authorities have been gradually formalising and standardising their approach to and encouragement of this option.

However, such placements are not without challenges and kinship carers and the children placed with them can need high levels of support, which may not be forthcoming. Some of the explanation for the patchy, and sometimes lack of support lies in the range of formal and informal routes into kinship care and the complexities surrounding the legal status of the children. In some instances, children may be "looked after" by the Local Authority while in others they are not. These differences in status and the attendant differences in entitlements to support from the Local authority can be very hard for Kinship carers to understand and to navigate their way through.

After years of campaigning by Family Rights Group, the Kinship Care Alliance and others for authorities to recognise and consistently provide support for family and friends carers, in 2011 the government issued long-awaited guidance to local authorities on family and friends care (DfE 2011). This statutory guidance "aims to improve outcomes for children and young people who, because they are unable to live with their parents, are being brought up by members of their extended families, friends or other people who are connected with them. In particular it provides guidance on the implementation of the duties in the Children Act 1989 in respect of such children and young people"(DfE 2011).

The guidance required authorities with responsibility for Children's Services to publish, by 30 September 2011, the authority's policy and approach towards supporting the needs of all children living with kinship carers, regardless of their legal status, and explains what the policy should cover. It states that:

- Policies should be underpinned by the principle that support should be based on the needs of the child rather than merely their legal status. (Para 4.6, pp 21-22)
- Children and young people who are unable to live with their parents should receive the support that they and their carers need to safeguard and promote their welfare, whether or not they are looked after. (Para 1.2, p 5)

It is too soon to judge what difference the guidance is making but the crucial test will be how soon and how well it translates into changes in services and practice, as experienced by children and the family and friends carers they live with.

It is unlikely that the picture of "patchy" support will change dramatically in the short term, especially given the current context of constrained budgets and general retrenchment. It is imperative therefore that kinship care is given continuous strategic focus and attention by Local Authorities, and that there is external challenge to services to ensure that policies are implemented and improvements secured and sustained.

The Oxford University and Family Rights Group study *"Kinship Care, Legal status and support"*, due to be published later in 2012, will give some good insights into the experiences of children and family or friends carers and of the steps needed to support effective implementation of the guidance.

Crossover posts

Some local authorities have created 'crossover posts', where an individual member of staff's role is to provide and enable a link between two different services whose work remit overlaps. Such workers are usually based within one or other of the teams primarily, while being significantly involved in the other team's work; for example, a mental health worker or substance misuse worker based in a children and families team or vice versa.

The role of such workers varies, with some taking on case responsibility for families with overlapping needs; others providing an advisory role; and others helping to set up systems and collect information on the numbers of children or parents affected by dual issues locally. Some are also involved in the training or development of other staff. Below there is a more detailed description of the role of one such worker, providing insight into the scope of the role. Another person in a crossover post on the project had a development role, highlighting unmet need to senior management and producing a joint working protocol.

Such workers are well placed to see how current systems, procedures and arrangements are working, so it is essential that they are well supported and that what they learn through their unique vantage point is fed into wider service planning. Also, being in lone posts such as these can be very challenging so it is essential to have good supervision and to make links with others in similar roles in other services.

Whilst these posts represent a positive step, and demonstrate an increasing recognition by services of the need for a more joined-up approach, they are perhaps best seen as a short-term measure, with the long-term aim being to establish effective joint working arrangements and confident skilled practitioners across the range of services. Reliance on one worker or post to fill such a gap needs to be tempered with a recognition of its limitations – potentially too much pressure on one person and the likelihood that locating the expertise and knowledge in one person will mean much of it will go when they leave the service.

The 2003 SCIE report *Families That Have Alcohol and Mental Health Problems: A template for partnership working* (Kearney and others), provides further information and pointers about how such posts can be set up and utilised.

User involvement

Improving the effectiveness of parental and family support services depends on listening and responding to previous and current service users' experiences, views and ideas about those services. Statutory and voluntary services have increasingly become aware of the value, and indeed the necessity (if services are to be truly responsive), of enabling children's participation in decisions affecting them and in facilitating the involvement of adult service users in service development.

The extent to which such involvement and consultation occurs meaningfully in practice is variable between agencies and there is still much that can be done. The Social Care Institute for Excellence, for example, identified the importance of user involvement in developing joint working protocols, but there is little evidence of this happening on any large scale. In the work being done to create greater partnership between commissioner and provider agencies and towards more integrated working, however, consultation with parents, children and the wider community about their concerns, experiences and needs are an essential element.

Where service users have been meaningfully involved, the benefits can be a greater sense of ownership of the services by users, greater engagement, increased accessibility, flexibility, improved communication and, not least, more effective services that are more likely to achieve their desired outcomes.

There is potential for service users (adults and children) to enhance the quality of services at all stages from initial identification of needs and service gaps through to service development, delivery, evaluation and review.

Service users can be involved in service provision on the macro level (for example in protocol development or helping map needs and gaps geographically across areas); or at the micro level (for example introducing more choice and involvement in individual packages of support, for individual users or families, including encouraging professional flexibility in terms of where workers meet clients). Direct payment arrangements are one lever for increasing user choice at the individual level, although it is important that appropriate support is provided to recipients and professionals to ensure this process is workable and helpful. In the DfES guidance, *Joint Planning and Commissioning Framework for Children, Young People and Maternity Services* (2006), Trafford is given as a practice example. It makes 'options funding' – a sum of money from which services can be purchased – available to young people to be spent in consultation with them as a means of encouraging greater choice, control and flexibility.

Participation or user involvement can take many forms and can provide different levels of involvement and service user control. Consultations tend to be one-off processes – gaining the views of adult or children service users on a particular issue, service or draft plan. Methods range from group meetings or one-to-one interviews, to paper, email or web-based questionnaires. Sometimes large scale events, to which a wide range of potentially affected groups are invited, are used as a way of gaining diverse views; they can also be used as forums for electing service user representatives. Advisory and steering groups are another mechanism for drawing in the expertise and opinions of service users to inform the running of services or projects.

On the macro level of service development, service users may become members of committees or elected as trustees. Parallel structures (bodies set up to shadow organisational committees that provide feedback to those bodies on decisions and plans) are sometimes set up. On the micro level, formal mechanisms are useful for obtaining feedback from service users about services or interventions as they occur, or soon after they occur; for reviewing progress; and, when collated, for informing the service as a whole about users' views and the effectiveness of the support provided.

Participants on the Building Resilience project had various experiences of participation and user involvement within their own services. They emphasised the importance of user feedback being put into concrete action, as even the most empowering-seeming model could otherwise be merely tokenistic. It takes time and requires commitment by all involved to evolve a good level of active participation.

Before involving service users in service activities, it is helpful to focus on clarifying what the expectations are in terms of what it is hoped will be achieved and whether this is realistic. At what stage will service users be involved and how will that involvement be resourced? What will participating service users get out of it and how will feedback will be shared and responded to?

One of the greatest challenges is finding ways to ensure that user involvement processes get at views that are *truly* representative. Nearly all agencies participating in the project reported that, in their local areas, it tended to be the same group of parents, often the most vocal, who provided the 'user voice' – when in fact they shared little in common with 'harder to reach' groups (for example parents with mental health problems or those with substance misuse issues) who were rarely involved.

Factors that ensured that such views and experiences were canvassed were those designed to check that processes were in place at the time users were receiving services. These were, for example:

- regular reviews
- facilitated discussions
- semi-structured interviews.

Also helpful in specifically targeting marginalised groups are one-to-one opportunities for users to give their views confidentially (rather than where groups are invited, as this situation can inhibit many people). Attention to physical access issues, help with transport and child care, and ensuring the environment in which consultation activities take place is comfortable and 'neutral' (that is, not the same building in which child protection conferences may have taken place, for example) are all important aspects of planning. Finally, using accessible language and ensuring adequate feedback of what has been found and what will happen as a result are essential.

When done well, service user involvement adds meaning and value to a service. Whilst many organisations have 'user-involvement' or 'participation workers' or commission these tasks from specialist agencies, it is important that responsibility for accessing and utilising service user feedback is owned by everyone within a service. The user represents the service and it is essentially everyone's responsiveness and openness that will determine how service users view the service – and therefore how inclined they will be to enter into a dialogue that occurs naturally and in an ongoing, more immediate way.

Training and skills development

As discussed earlier, the dominance of 'single user' agencies in which staff are trained and skilled in working with either the child, adolescent, parent or carer means there is a lack of expertise and confidence for many in having a whole-family approach. It is understandable that adult mental health workers often lack confidence in talking to children or in being able to give a view about 'parenting capacity', for example. However, an increase in the awareness of all relevant professionals about the impact family members have on each other is essential. Similarly, it is necessary to have an increased understanding of the possible implications of professional interventions, or the lack of them, on the family members of the service user.

It is not realistic or necessary for all professionals to be 'expert' in all aspects of family life and circumstances, but it is necessary for professionals to have some awareness of key issues and to know 'what each other knows' and when and how to tap into this knowledge. It is also necessary for practitioners to be able to think beyond the limitations of a 'service led' approach, which can come from rigid eligibility thresholds and service boundaries. Even if professionals don't know how, or if, they are in a position to respond to the knock-on needs within a family, a failure to recognise and report such needs appropriately is dangerous.

The extent to which formal training can address this is debatable, but it certainly has an important part to play. Forrester and Harwin (2006) argue for better training and more input on substance misuse on the social work degree course to better reflect the prevalence of such issues in social work caseloads. Participants on the Building Resilience project commented that they tended to receive one-off training days on 'mental health' or 'drug awareness' or 'child protection'. However, many thought that if such training could be built up so that there was the opportunity to learn further, at an increasing level, it would be preferable.

Interagency or joint training can be positive and can increase understanding of professional roles and the scope for complementing each other's work. However, this is most effective when such training is preceded by and builds on clear joint working arrangements or protocols. However, training is not the only, or necessarily the most effective, way of enhancing knowledge and skills and the informal learning that can occur through joint working is invaluable. Making formal arrangements for staff to visit and 'shadow' the work of other professionals, or setting up secondments between services, can be a very useful way forward to enhance the development of staff in both services. Thorough staff inductions, which allow enough time for workers to get to grips with both their own organisation and the other relevant services (preferably through visits) are also important.

Some resources for training and team development that may help enhance the knowledge, skills or awareness of professionals in their work with parental mental health or substance misuse are referred to in the Further resources section.

Practice example 9 shows how adult mental health workers identified and addressed their knowledge and skills gaps through training in order to enable them to consider children's needs.

Practice example 9: Tower Hamlets

Home Treatment Team

Breaking down barriers between adult mental health and children's services; and helping a Home Treatment Team talk about parenting.

The multidisciplinary Home Treatment Team in Tower Hamlets, part of the East London Foundation Trust, has made significant strides in recognising the impact of mental illness on parenting and on children. This is in line with Trust policy on safeguarding children, and raised expectations within the Trust that workers will not only identify risk to children but also identify their wider emotional and developmental needs, while supporting the adults in their role as parents. This has led to some anxiety and questions from staff who requested additional teaching input.

Staff identified their concerns and confusion about matters such as sharing information, making a referral to children and families services, or routinely notifying children and family services of mental health services' involvement. These tasks created extra pressure for a team whose involvement with a family is likely to be brief. Disclosing information to another agency was thought to conflict with codes of practice and professional ethics. The main anxiety seemed to lie in raising the matter at all with someone who may be very unwell. Staff were uncomfortable with the idea of telling a service user, who may be already acutely embarrassed by the need for mental health services involvement, that they needed to inform or involve yet another agency. Staff were also unclear about whether there would be any benefit to the family of such actions.

The team invited the Coordinator for Children in Families with Mental Illness, who works across adult mental health and children's services, to plan two workshops with them to help them find ways of managing these responsibilities in a way that they, as well as the service user, could feel comfortable with.

For the first of these the coordinator invited the Trust's Safeguarding Children nurse advisor, and social workers from the Children and Families Advice and Assessment team, to clarify policy and referral procedures. The whole team participated in an informal quiz, and had the opportunity to ask questions of the other service. Staff discovered that they knew more than they had previously thought, clarified points of confusion, and became more realistic in their expectations of the other service, and respectful of each service's workloads. Differences of language, terminology and statutory framework were sorted out.

The second workshop focused on how to talk to families when one had concerns about children, and the coordinator was joined by a CAMHS family therapist as co-facilitator. Through discussion and role-play, staff revealed deeper fears and anxieties but were also able to learn from each other and come up with a comprehensive list of good practice points.

Some of the fears expressed were about:

- facing the user's hostility
- breaking the therapeutic relationship and creating distrust
- increasing stigma
- impinging on civil liberties
- going against culturally prevalent behaviours – including what is appropriate in the worker's own culture
- making someone more ill by adding to existing stress
- creating fears that they would lose the children
- betraying the user
- obtaining 'permission to share information' then telling the whole world
- following procedure just because the political climate had changed.

Several workers reported that talking to families about the impact of the illness on their children was not a problem; and, indeed, that to confront a client with the reality of the damage they might be causing to family relationships, and the likely consequences, could be a helpful therapeutic step.

The learning points, which emerged from the discussion, were that it was important to:

- feel clear and confident in your role and in what you are saying
- remain calm and matter of fact
- avoid jargon or legalistic language
- be transparent and fill in any forms together with the service user

- be positive about what might be gained from contacting children's services, and from services working together
- recognise and acknowledge the support already available within the family
- pick up on the user's own concerns or wishes for help
- take care with timing and wait, unless there is an urgent situation, until the user's mental state allows them to listen and take in what is being said.

During the workshop, the team were able to make positive use of their own varied experiences to identify good practice points and to learn from each other. There was increased confidence in what was possible, and on the strengths of working together. Now participants are back at work, they report that they feel less anxious when discussing children's well-being with families, and are able to present interventions in a more positive light. They have increased confidence when using their own initiative to liaise with schools and other children's services, with the families' agreement; and thinking about children is built into daily practice.

Jemma Clarke-Cooper, Judith Edwards, Emma Hunt, Peter Joseph, Rosemary Loshak, Lorette McQueen, Philip Myers

For further information contact:
Rosemary Loshak, Coordinator for Children in Families with Mental Illness
7th Floor Anchorage House, 2 Clove Crescent, London E14 2BE
Rosie.Loshak@towerhamlets.gov.uk or Lorette.McQueen@elcmht.nhs.uk

Increased capacity to involve fathers

The tendency for services to fail to include or engage with fathers successfully through assessment and provision of support services is well documented. This can be seen in part as being due to wider staffing and recruitment issues, as most of the workforce is female. Whilst this needs addressing, there need to be more proactive attempts through the design of services to make them more accessible and inclusive.

> Men think 'Well this service isn't for me' so basically they don't have very high expectations of it. Wherever a service does engage fathers, they find that they are enthusiastic recipients of the service. Most men if you engage with them about parenting, will be so surprised that anyone is talking to them that they are grateful for anything

> (National Voluntary Organisation (DfES 2006b, p.33))

Ghate and others (2000) examined some of the barriers that reduced fathers' likelihood of accessing Children's Centre and SureStart programme-based support. Their feedback can be seen to be relevant to a far wider range of services. The barriers were listed as:

- policies and priorities that assume 'parents' to be synonymous with mothers
- referral systems that are geared towards mothers and children inconvenient opening hours
- lack of male staff and staff unsure how to interact with men due to being more used to women accessing the service
- 'feminised atmosphere'
- family centres perceived as a place of refuge for women
- women outnumbering men/lack of male presence some women were perceived as unfriendly, unwelcoming or even overtly hostile towards men

- activities – such as sitting drinking coffee, watching children play, talking with other parents, and aromatherapy – that were seen as 'female' and not enjoyed by men
- a perceived willingness in staff to engage with mothers as women as well as parents, but not fathers as men
- cultural ones, that is, some centres were offering services to Muslim women where including men would be inappropriate.

They found that the factors that enabled men's involvement within such services were:

- referral-only centres or parts of centres – because men tended to stick more closely to programmes of involvement when they had formally been referred to centres (although some doubt existed as to whether fathers got engaged with the centre in any more than a superficial way)
- management attitudes that were seen as objective, not biased towards mothers, and that involved actively encouraging fathers
- male workers (male facilitators of groups and activities were particularly important)
- a willingness of staff to build relationships with fathers on their own terms and often away from the family centre
- staff persistence
- referral systems targeted at both mothers and fathers
- a less hostile atmosphere – for example, the presence of other men or male staff, and a welcoming building
- activities that men saw as more 'male', such as those related to DIY, and BBQs, parties and other types of social family-oriented events.

Some services such as substance misuse services are more experienced in working with men individually and in groups (Morris and Wates 2006). It is worth services that struggle with this finding out more about the structures and models of service provision that such services have adopted that seem to be successful in engaging men with the services. Family Group Conferences are another model within children's services that have been successful in involving fathers.

> It requires going out there because you have to overcome a cultural thing. A service to get there needs to be proactive. A lot of services say 'We are for everyone but fathers don't come.' It's the responsibility of the service. It's about targeting. There are lots of ways for targeting. It's where you market. Generally programmes find that you have to go to where the fathers are – you have to go to them – pubs, sports clubs, employers. Employment agencies. You have to organise activities that men feel comfortable with

> (National Voluntary Organisation (DfES 2006b, p.33))

Black and minority ethnic groups: Promoting more accessible services

If service planners and those delivering services are to reduce the barriers to accessibility for black and minority ethnic groups, they will need to make significant change. Concerns about a lack of resources and skills to bring about such changes often lead to compromise. It is a highly complex task to meet the differing needs of a variety of BME communities in the same locality; and a 'one size fits all' approach is inappropriate and will simply compound difficulties. However, as with reducing stigma more generally, it is in everyone's interests to overcome these problems. The likely solutions, such as community inclusion – enabling BME groups and organisations to take forward the design and delivery of parenting services (suggested by the DfES (2006b) research to be the most widely agreed effective strategy) – fit well with the wider moves and agendas towards greater community and voluntary sector engagement in social and health care provision that are already underway.

Establishing an ethnically diverse workforce, which is more representative of the communities it is there to serve, is a challenge for workforce development initiatives. Additionally, the existing workforce requires support in becoming more 'culturally capable' – as recommended by the Race Equality Action plan. The current picture of race-related training is patchy and fragmented, with no agreed definition of 'cultural competence'. However, Joanne Bennet from the Sainsbury Centre for Mental Health (in Lyall 2006) found in her review of training that there is currently a lack of evidence that such race-related training works in producing better services. She argues that it is more important to look at structural processes and power relationships in the way services are delivered. Cultural competence training in the police, following the Lawrence inquiry, had no effect according to Richard Stone (a panel member of the Lawrence and Bennet inquiries) (in Lyall 2006).

Training and awareness raising that is planned and delivered by or in conjunction with service users seems to be more effective. The East London and City Mental Health Trust held a focus group with service users, scriptwriters and staff and created a play to raise awareness of service user views, needs and experiences. Evaluation of the impact of this on the over 100 mental health staff who saw the play showed that they had an improved awareness of discrimination and many talked afterwards of the need to improve their listening skills as a result (Lyall 2006).

Responses

At the same time, assumptions that particular groups are 'hard to reach' should be avoided. The government's Delivering Race Equality in Mental Health Care: An action plan for reform inside and outside services (Department of Health 2005) recommended that Primary Care Trusts appoint 500 community workers to help develop services to black and minority ethnic communities and proposed that funding be made available for community engagement programmes and training (Lyall 2006). Such initiatives, along with moves towards greater community and voluntary group engagement in local planning, represent opportunities to improve the accessibility of services to all.

Other elements of improving access involve carrying out needs assessment of local BME communities and planning services with an explicit recognition of some of the barriers to access.

Promoting more effective professional responses to stigma

There can be a tendency for stigma to be seen as something inevitable that cannot be changed (Thornicroft 2006). This view can understandably lead services to view it as out of their control and remit. However, the impacts on those affected, who come into contact with services (or who don't come into contact but may need support), is very much within the remit of services. Supporting people in managing the impact on them of stigma can help promote their overall well-being and recovery; is a vital part of any holistic assessment of needs; and can help prevent difficulties from worsening and necessitating more extreme forms of intervention. The SEU do not underestimate its significance.

> *Stigma and discrimination can affect people long after the symptoms of mental health problems have been resolved. Discrimination can lead to relapses in mental health problems and can intensify existing symptoms.*

> (Link and others 1997)

However, not only is there a need for the relevant services to support people with the impact of stigma and discrimination, but also to ensure that services themselves are not the source of discrimination; treating people unfairly or denying them opportunities. A widespread recognition and adoption of a social model of disability is an important basis for change. Such a model reduces the tendency to locate the problem within the individual, instead it focuses on addressing disabling barriers, including negative attitudes and unequal access (Morris and Wates 2006). Currently, few interventions address the significant structural and social factors that affect the life outcomes for this group of families, despite previous research clearly identifying the need to do so (Fraser and others 2006).

In the case of mental health, the Disability Discrimination Act (2005) is one route by which discriminating factors can be diminished if it is proactively applied. Also programmes aimed at tackling stigma now place more emphasis on discrimination, thereby focusing on society's response rather than placing the onus on the presence of mental health issues.

Services can do more to raise awareness locally about some of these issues among staff through a consistent reinforcement of anti-discriminatory principles within policies, protocols, training and management emphasis, as well as by giving information. Such awareness raising can and should extend beyond the internal range of an organisation, as those with unique service perspectives and specialist knowledge are well placed to educate and raise the awareness of others.

Another way in which stigma will be eroded is through service user involvement and collaboration in the planning and delivery of training, service provision and monitoring of effectiveness of services. It seems logical that those best placed to dispel assumptions and myths are those who are the subject of them. Also, attitudes and behaviours towards 'different' groups of people improve by spending more time with them according to 'contact hypothesis' (Allport 1954).

Examples of user involvement in reducing stigma are provided by Thornicroft (2006). A project run in London by Rethink and the Institute of Psychiatrists involves organising and delivering lectures and role-play sessions (in conjunction with service users) for medical students and those training to be psychiatrists in order to combat stigma. This is based on work in Kent, where school pupils and police were shown to have less stigmatising attitudes after they received awareness raising sessions from service users.

95

Evaluation

There is a body of knowledge and evidence about the impact of parental mental health problems on children and families, but less has been done to identify 'what works' in supporting parenting in these circumstances. Similarly, there is some research regarding the long-term impact of parental alcohol misuse and less on parental drug misuse but less still on what interventions help (both with these issues and more generally in promoting resilience, see Fraser and others 2006). For those approaches that are being tried and shared with others, both for their own effectiveness and as a practice model for others, it is necessary to evaluate them. Unfortunately there is currently a lack of evaluated practice approaches, so this is of particular importance.

Evaluation can be described as systematic planned activities, which take place in order to assess the effectiveness or outcomes of a service or project.

As well as providing an evidence base for determining 'what works' and what doesn't and enabling others to replicate promising approaches, evaluation is also necessary for demonstrating the 'worth' of a project to stakeholders or potential funders.

Evaluation can elicit useful information about the 'process' of the service activity or intervention or about its 'outcomes'. Shaw (2005a) sets out ten stages in a 'process overview chart' within her Evaluation Toolkit and stresses the importance of going through each one.

Process Overview

1 **Embarking on evaluation** – establishing why one is doing it, who for and how it will be used

2 **What kind of evaluation?** – considering types and styles of approach and what is appropriate, ethical, affordable and who might be involved

3 **Framing evaluation questions** – asking what do you want to find out/need to know or demonstrate? Ensuring you have SMART (Specific, Measurable, Attainable, Realistic, Time-based) questions

4 **Evaluation design** – deciding how to get at the evidence needed and choosing the approach and design

5 **Selecting methods** – selecting or designing the tools or instruments needed to carry out the evaluation

Before moving on from here, review steps 2, 3, 4 and 5. Can it be more efficient; and are the chosen methods and preferred style compatible?

6 **Detailed planning** – agreeing a plan and timetable for what will happen and when

7 **Data collection in progress** – taking steps to minimise any bias that you identify as potentially occurring in the data

Review and make any adjustments as necessary

8 **Making sense of your data** – organising, summarising and collating the data/findings

9 **Communication and dissemination** – informing relevant stakeholders; considering how, when, and in what form to do this

10 **Reflecting on the process and using the findings** – consider making changes to your practice or service and any ideas for future evaluation or research.

> Shaw, C (2005, 2nd Edition) *Nifty Evaluation: An introductory handbook for social care staff with a rough guide to evaluation resources.* Research in Practice in partnership with NCB, London

All too often the first and last two steps are not given enough attention, which hinders the usefulness of evaluation activities and wastes time and energy. When done well, evaluation forms the basis of service improvement.

7. Conclusion

Chapter 1 of this handbook highlighted that parental substance misuse and parental mental health problems affect a substantial portion of the population as a whole and in particular those who come into contact with services. There is an urgent and essential need for services to respond effectively to the needs of families affected by these issues because, while their presence does not necessarily result in adverse outcomes for children, it often does, and the impact on them can be serious and long lasting.

An examination of the potential impact of such family circumstances on children in Chapter 2 demonstrates that there is a lack of research into families who are coping well and that most research is focused on mothers rather than fathers. The research that is available mainly concerns families who come into contact with services and illustrates that they have an increased likelihood of experiencing poverty, poor housing, stigma and isolation.

The ability of parents to ensure their children's safety and provide boundaries, stimulation, physical care, supervision, consistency and routines can be significantly impeded. For children, this can have a cumulative impact that is detrimental to their physical and mental health. They may develop emotional and behavioural difficulties; experience reduced integration and success in their education; and may adopt coping strategies that are not necessarily positive. Many children become young carers, adding to the challenges they face and the sense of responsibility they may feel. Where parents struggle to show emotional warmth to their children due to their changing moods or presentation this can affect children's self-esteem and ability to form relationships, as can the secrecy and stigma often experienced by children in these circumstances.

Less often, children can be at risk of abuse or serious neglect that could be fatal (for example where dangerous substances are accessible to children) or at least significantly harmful. There is increasing recognition of the impact of neglect on children of all ages including adolescents. At the same time, the potential risks to children can increase for very young children or babies; when mental health problems are psychotic in nature or parental delusions involve the child; when domestic violence is present; or when substance misuse is coupled with mental ill-health.

Broader research into 'resilience' (discussed in Chapter 3) indicates that the presence of certain 'protective factors' are associated with better outcomes and increased resilience for children and families. These protective factors include a supportive partner; accessible and non-stigmatising community resources; a stable trustworthy adult within or outside the extended family who takes a consistent interest in a child's life; supportive social networks; and the opportunity to achieve, build self-esteem and maintain important family rituals and routines.

In order to safeguard children and to support families in better meeting their needs, it is essential that professional responses are based both on a good understanding of the day-to-day experience of children and the actual or likely impact on the developing child of any specific unmet needs or risks that are present, alongside a good understanding of the family's experiences and needs. Generalisations and value judgements need to be guarded against and, where possible, the positive aspirations of family members, their motivation for change and strengths need to be recognised and harnessed to support better outcomes. An increased understanding of the importance of protective factors among families, and the professionals who work with them, could empower people to influence and nurture the positives and strengths, perhaps leading to better outcomes.

If children cannot safely remain within their immediate family, timely and robust decisions need to made about their future. This should be based on a sound understanding of individual circumstances and a thorough exploration of whether or not the provision of appropriate support could ameliorate the situation within the timescale appropriate to the child's needs. Throughout this handbook the point has been made that the provision of appropriate support is sometimes lacking and that there is often scope for professional responses to be more focused, coordinated and therefore more effective.

There are a number of reasons for this. Relevant legislation and policy (discussed in Chapter 1 and Appendix 2) tend to be fragmented, often failing to recognise adult service users as parents and the impact that individual family members have on one another. Furthermore, the structure of 'single-user' services militates against a 'family focus'. Resource constraints lead to high thresholds for services and limited support being on offer. As a result, despite the goodwill and rhetoric about preventive services and more integrated working, statutory services tend to be reactive, inaccessible and not joined up in their approach. Outcomes for families are poor, with only half of 'problem drug-using' parents known to services having their children still living with them. Interventions tend to occur late and at 'the heavy end'. For the many more children adversely affected by parental alcohol use there is a tendency for under-intervention or for significant delays in decision-making. For those affected by parental mental health problems, there is little support when mental health problems are classed as 'mild' or 'moderate' even though the impact on the child can still be significant.

Other hindrances to good practice in this area are discussed in Chapter 4. They indicate a need for more collaborative, analytical assessments and decision-making and an increase in knowledge and awareness among adults' and children's practitioners. Other obstacles include the challenge of engaging with resistant service users or those who fear services; along with practical barriers, for example a lack of family-friendly facilities within traditionally 'adult' services such as psychiatric hospitals or drug services.

Chapter 5 explored some of the ways in which practice can better support families. It included the need for training and skills development; and for more focused whole-family support (underpinned by clear assessments) that is helpful to children and parents practically and emotionally. This, and the need for information and support to informal networks, is well documented but still far from being sufficiently available.

At the strategic level (discussed in Chapter 6), there is clearly a need for improved data collection and analysis (to enhance a local understanding of prevalence and enable resources to be targeted more appropriately). There is also a need to gain more qualitative information, through carrying out an ongoing evaluation of services with service users relating their experiences and needs. Financial constraints are difficult to influence but there is scope for maximising the funding and resources available.

An examination of the strategic changes necessary to enable services to better respond to parental mental health or parental substance use illustrates a much wider issue. There is a need for more integrated, family-focused services across the board, in all circumstances where individual needs impact on families as a whole. It is likely that many suggestions made within this handbook, about strategic and practice issues, will be relevant to working with other families with complex needs.

To enable relevant professionals to 'think family', there needs to be a clear message coming from senior levels of organisations that safeguarding children is everybody's responsibility. This needs to be supported by clear expectations about working; backed up by protocols, training and coherent policies in related areas such as dual diagnosis and kinship care. Organisations need to be proactive in increasing the accessibility of their services to black and minority ethnic families, to fathers and to other potential service users who may anticipate that services will be discriminatory towards them.

Finally, it is important to acknowledge that there is much good work already being undertaken with individuals and with families and there is a wealth of knowledge, skills and positive motivation within the children and adult's services workforce. To support this further, a culture of collaboration and joint working, even informally 'picking each other's brains' when thresholds are not met, along with an openness to learn from each other and from service users, can only be beneficial for service users and practitioners alike.

Further resources

Below is an alphabetical list of relevant organisations – with website addresses included as sources of additional relevant information. A few relevant books, videos and training packages are also listed.

Organisations and their websites

Adfam

http://www.adfam.org.uk

Provides telephone advice, website information and services for families affected by alcohol and drug misuse. It has also produced the following publications.

Bouncing Back! Creative learning pack for work with families, available from Adfam website price £15..

We Count Too – published by three family-support organisations: Adfam, Pada and Famfed. These are good practice guides for those working with family members affected by someone else's drug use. Available online at www.drugs.gov.uk

Adfam
25 Corsham Street
London
N1 6DR
Tel: 020 7553 7640
Fax: 020 7253 7991
admin@adfam.org.uk

Alcohol Concern

http://www.alcoholconcern.org.uk

Provides information on services, factsheets on alcohol, and a helpline.

It provides, through a separate website (below), toolkits for supporting children and parents, called *Alcohol and families*. The toolkit includes information on supporting parents; training and resources; resilience and multi-agency working; and guidance for professionals, including a toolkit for teachers.

www.alcoholandfamilies.org.uk

Alcohol Concern
Suite B5 West Wing
New City Cloisters
196 Old Street
London EC1V 9FR
Tel: 020 7566 9800

Barnardo's

http://www.barnardos.org.uk

Produces publications, including free downloads; practitioner resources; young carers projects, and more.

Barnardo's
Tanners Lane
Barkingside
Ilford
Essex
IG6 1QG
Tel: 020 8550 8822
Fax: 020 8551 6870

The Centre for Excellence and Outcomes in Children and Young People's Services (C4EO)

www.c4eo.org.uk

The Centre for Excellence and Outcomes in Children and Young People's Services provides a range of products and support services to improve outcomes. For the first time, excellence in local practice, combined with national research and data about 'what works' is being gathered in one place. C4EO shares this evidence and the best of local practice with all those who work with and for children and young people and provides practical 'hands on support' to help local areas make full use of this evidence.

One of its key work themes is Families, Parents and Carers – Improving the safety, health and wellbeing of children through improving the physical and mental health of mothers, fathers and carers.

C4EO
8 Wakley Street
London
EC1V 7QE
Switchboard: 020 7843 6358
Email: contactus@c4eo.org.uk

ChildLine

www.childline.org.uk

Is the free national helpline for children and young people in danger and distress. It provides a confidential counselling service for any child with any problem 24 hours a day, every day. It listens, comforts and protects. Trained counsellors provide support and advice and can refer children in danger to appropriate helping agencies.

NSPCC
Weston House
42 Curtain Road
London
EC2A 3NH
0800 1111 (helpline)

The Children's Society

www.childrenssociety.org.uk

Supports the STARS Project, a national initiative providing information and support for children and young people whose parents misuse drugs/alcohol. The contact details for the STARS Project are:

0115 942 2974
www.starsnationalinitiative.org.uk

Children of Addicted Parents and People

www.coap.co.uk

A self-help website for young people to discuss their concerns about a person who is abusing drugs or alcohol.

Care Quality Commission

www.cqc.org.uk

Runs a website that includes information for service users, carers, children and professionals. Information is available in different languages.

CQC National Customer Service Centre
Citygate
Newcastle NE1 4PA
Tel: 03000 616161

Dartington Social Research Unit

www.dartington.org.uk

Dartington Social Research Unit undertake and report on research regarding children in need, child development and children's services.

Dartington Social Research Unit
Lower Hood Barn
Dartington
Devon
TQ9 6AB
Tel: 01803 762400
Fax: 01803 762983
unit@dartington.org.uk

Department for Education

www.education.gov.uk

Information includes research, statistics and data for professionals and families.

DFE
Castle View House
East Lane
Runcorn
Cheshire WA7 2GJ
Tel: 0370 0002288
Typetalk 18001 0370 0002288, contact also through website.

Department of Health

http://www.dh.gov.uk

Provides health and social care policy, guidance and publications.

Information about alcohol misuse and substance misuse can be accessed on this site.

Department of Health
Richmond House
79 Whitehall
London SW1A 2NS
Tel: 020 7210 4850
Text phone 020 7210 5025

Disabled Parents Network

www.DisabledParentsNetwork.org.uk

Produces reports and guidance for professionals and handbooks to support disabled parents, their families and those working with them.

0300 3300 639 (general enquiries)
information@disabledparentsnetwork.org.uk

DrugScope

http://www.drugscope.org.uk

Is an independent centre of expertise on drugs, informing policy development and reducing drug-related risk. The website includes information and DrugData database of drugs literature. The information is available in different languages. 'D World' is a drug-information website for 11–14-year-olds.

DrugScope
Prince Consort House
Suite 204 (2nd Floor)
109/111 Farringdon Road
London
EC1R 3BW
Tel: 020 7520 7550
Fax: 020 7520 7555
info@drugscope.org.uk

Family Rights Group

www.frg.org.uk

Provides advice and support for families whose children are involved with social services; and develops and promotes services that help secure the best possible futures for children and families. Has information on family and friends as carers and on family group conferencing. Has a range of publications, including ones aimed at and about kinship carers. Information on Family Group Conferences for policy makers, family members, managers, social workers, coordinators and anyone who may refer a family to, or attend, a family group conference (FGC).

Family Rights Group
Second Floor
The Print House
18 Ashwin Street
London
E8 3DL
Tel: 020 7923 2628
Fax: 020 7923 2683
office@frg.org.uk
Advice Line 0808 8010366
advice@frg.org.uk

Families Anonymous

www.familiesanonymous.org

Runs advice and support groups for families and friends who are concerned about the use of drugs or related behavioural problems. Literature also available.

Families Anonymous
Doddington and Rollo Community Association
Charlotte Despard Avenue
Battersea
London
SW11 5HD
Tel: 0845 1200 660 (helpline)
office@famanon.org.uk

Family Action (formerly Family Welfare Association (FWA))

www.family-action.org.uk

Provides home and project support for families, community-based mental health services and financial help for families. The website includes downloadable leaflets on services.

Family Action Central Office
501–505 Kingsland Road
London
E8 4AU
020 7254 6251

FRANK

www.talktofrank.com

Is a cross-departmental campaign, which is led by the Department of Health/Home Office. Provides information and free confidential advice services through a helpline; and information and advice about drugs, their consequences and supporting services, through a website and other resources. Frank information is still available on the website, although the website indicates that further development is suspended.

Tel: 0800 776600 24 hr.

Joseph Rowntree Foundation

www.jrf.org.uk

Is a social policy research and development charity. Its research themes include: housing, poverty, drugs and alcohol, and parenting. Website includes publications.

JRF (Head Office)
The Homestead
40 Water End
York YO30 6WP
Tel 01904 629241
info@jrf.org.uk

Lifeline

www.lifeline.org.uk

Provides services for families affected by drug/alcohol misuse. Produces a range of publications about drugs and drug use.

Head office
Lifeline Project Ltd
39-41 Thames St
Manchester M4 1NA
Tel 0161 8347160

Mind

www.mind.org.uk

Is a mental health charity covering England and Wales. It is involved in:

- advancing the views, needs and ambitions of people with mental health problems
- challenging discrimination and promoting inclusion
- influencing policy through campaigning and education
- inspiring the development of quality services which reflect expressed need and diversity
- achieving equal rights through campaigning and education.

0300 1233393 (information line)
info@mind.org.uk

NACOA

www.nacoa.org.uk

Is the abbreviation for National Association of Children of Alcoholics, which was founded to provide information, advice and support for children of alcoholics and people concerned for their welfare. Leaflets for children and parents are available as downloads.

0800 358 3456 (a free confidential helpline)
helpline@Nacoa.org.uk

Nacro

www.nacro.org.uk

The crime reduction charity, aims to make society safer by finding practical solutions to reducing crime. Since 1966 Nacro has worked to give ex-offenders, disadvantaged people and deprived communities the help they need to build a better future.

Head office
NACRO
Park Place
10-12 Lawn Lane
London SW8 1UD
Tel 0207 840 7200

National Children's Bureau (NCB)

www.ncb.org.uk

The National Children's Bureau is a leading research and development charity working to improve the lives of children and young people, reducing the impact of inequalities. NCB works with children, for children to influence government policy, be a strong voice for young people and front-line professionals, and provide practical solutions on a range of social issues.

Provides information on policy, research and best practice for professionals. Website includes information on publications (some downloadable) and current projects.

National Children's Bureau (NCB)
8 Wakley Street
London
EC1V 7QE
Tel: 020 7843 6000
Fax: 020 7278 9512
library@ncb.org.uk

National Drugs Helpline

Is a 24-hour, seven-days-a-week, free and confidential telephone service that offers advice and information for those who are concerned, or have questions, about drugs. The service is available to anyone.

0800 77 66 00

National Mental Health Development Unit (NMHDU)

www.nmhdu.org.uk

This unit closed in 2011, however publications and resources are still available to download from the website.

National Society for the Prevention of Cruelty to Children (NSPCC)

www.nspcc.org.uk

Provides direct services to children and families and campaigns to promote children's safety and well-being. Also produces publications, research and provides an information service.

There is an NSPCC Helpline for anyone concerned about a child – 0800 800 5000; ChildLine for children to obtain confidential advice and support – 0800 1111; and an interactive website for children and young people to discuss and seek advice on issues that concern them, www.childline.org.uk.

NSPCC
42 Curtain Road
London
EC2A 3NH

National Treatment Agency for Substance Misuse (NTA)

www.nta.nhs.uk

Is a special health authority, created by the government in 2001, to improve the availability, capacity and effectiveness of treatment for drug misuse in England. It is there to ensure that there is more treatment, better treatment and fairer treatment available to all those who need it. The website includes details of the NTA's work programme, as well as publications and guidance for those in the drug treatment sector and service users.

National Treatment Agency
6th Floor
Skipton House
80 London Road
London SE1 6LH
Tel: 0207 972 1999
nta.enquiries@nta-nhs.org.uk

Participation Works

www.participationworks.org.uk

Is based at the National Children's Bureau and is an online gateway to the world of children and young people's participation. The gateway provides a single access point to comprehensive information on policy, practice, networks, training and innovative ideas from across the UK.

Participation Works
8 Wakley Street
London
EC1V 7QE
Tel 0207 833 6815
enquiries@participationworks.org.uk

Research in Practice

www.rip.org.uk

Is the largest children and families research implementation project in England and Wales. Established in 1996, it is a department of The Dartington Hall Trust and is run in collaboration with the Association of Directors of Children's Services, The University of Sheffield and a network of over 100 participating agencies in the UK.

Its aims are to improve outcomes for vulnerable children and families in England and Wales by promoting and facilitating evidence-informed practice. The website provides news, views, research reviews, summaries, policy insights and information on projects and publications.

Research in Practice Social Justic Programme
The Granary
Dartington Hall
Totnes
Devon TQ9 6EQ
Tel: 01803 867692
Fax: 01803 868816
ask@rip.org.uk

The Royal College of Psychiatrists

www.rcpsych.ac.uk

Is the professional and educational body for psychiatrists in the United Kingdom and the Republic of Ireland. It aims to promote mental health by setting standards and promoting excellence in mental health care; improving understanding through research and education; leading, representing, training and supporting psychiatrists; and working with patients, carers and their organisations. The website includes information on drugs/alcohol and mental illness.

The Royal College of Psychiatrists
17 Belgrave Square
London
SW1X 8PG
Tel: 020 7235 2351
Fax: 020 7245 1231

Centre for Mental Health

www.centreformentalhealth.org.uk

Works to improve the quality of life for people with mental health problems by influencing policy and practice in mental health services. The focus is mainly on criminal justice and employment, and broad mental health policy. The aims of the Centre are furthered through project work, research, publications and events.

The Centre for Mental Health
134–138 Borough High Street
London
SE1 1LB
Tel: 020 7827 8300
Fax: 020 7827 8369
contact@centreformentalhealth.org.uk

Social Care Institute for Excellence (SCIE)

www.scie.org.uk

Aims to improve the experience of people who use social care by developing and promoting knowledge about good practice in the sector. Using knowledge gathered from diverse sources and a broad range of people and organisations, it develops resources which are shared freely, supporting those working in social care and empowering service users. Its publications include:

SCIE Resource Guide 1. Families that have Alcohol and Mental Health Problems: A template for partnership working. Accessible from: www.scie.or.uk/publications/resourceguides/rg01.pdf

SCIE Report No 2. Alcohol Drug and Mental Health Problems: Working with families. Accessible from: www.scie.org.uk/publications/reports/report02.pdf

Social Care Institute for Excellence
Fifth Floor
2–4 Cockspur Street
London SW1Y 5BH
Tel: 020 7024 7650
info@scie.org.uk

Stella Project

www.avaproject.org.uk/our-projects/stella-project.aspx

Is a partnership between the Greater London Domestic Violence Project (GLDVP) and the Greater London Alcohol and Drug Alliance (GLADA). The GLDVP works to end domestic violence across the capital by supporting direct service providers and promoting joint working. The GLADA, established by the Mayor of London in 2002, is a strategic network of organisations and agencies concerned with the problems caused by drugs and alcohol in London. The Stella Project provides briefings, good practice guidance and toolkits.

Stella Project enquiries
Tel: 020 7549 0276

Start in Manchester

www.startmc.org.uk

Is an arts and mental health project. Its website provides information about the project and online art from adults with mental health issues. Start[mc] helps people to improve, maintain and protect their mental well-being through art and gardening. Service users are people recovering from a period of serious and long-term mental ill health, and want to use art to build confidence, self-esteem and practical life skills.

High Elms
Upper Park Road
Victoria Park
Manchester
M14 5RU
Tel: 0161 257 0675 ● 0161 257 0510 ● 0161 257 0696
Fax: 0161 225 9410

Substance Misuse Management in General Practice (SMMGP)

www.smmgp.co.uk

Is a network to support GPs and other members of the primary healthcare team who work with substance misuse.

SMMGP
c/o National Treatment Agency for Substance Misuse
6th Floor
Skipton House
80 London Road
London
SE1 6LH
smmgp@btinternet.com

Women's Aid

www.womensaid.org.uk

Provides information and help, including a 24-hour, national domestic violence helpline 0808 2000247.

Tel: 0117 944 4411 (general enquiries only)
Fax: 0117 924 1703
info@womensaid.org.uk

Books

When a Family is in Trouble: Children can cope with grief from drug and alcohol addiction
Marge Heegaard (1993) Woodland Press. ISBN 978-0962050275.

When Someone has a Very Serious Illness: Children can learn to cope with loss and change (drawing out feelings)
Marge Heegaard (1991) Woodland Press, ISBN 978-0962050244.

Different Like Me: A book for teens who worry about their parent's use of alcohol/drugs
Evelyn Leite and Pamela Espeland (1999) Hazelden Information and Educational Services, ISBN 978-0935908343.

Up and Down the Mountain: Helping children cope with parental alcoholism
Pamela L Higgins (1994) New Horizons Press. ISBN 978-0882821337.

NCB publications

Available from www.ncb.org.uk/books

Talking About Alcohol and Other Drugs: A guide for looked after children's services
Butcher, J and Ryan, M (2006) ISBN 1 904787 789.

For managers of looked after children's services, training managers, managers of children and young people's residential homes and social workers. 81 pages.

Adult Drug Problems, Children's Needs: Assessing the impact of parental drug use – a toolkit for practitioners
Hart, D and Powell, J (2007) ISBN 978 1904787976.

Provides a range of practice tools including checklists for: 'engagement and assessment', 'team managers' 'thinking about care planning' (which refers to when residential family placements should be considered, the need for plans to reflect children's needs and timescales, and twin-track planning), 'supporting kinship carers' and provides a checklist to use when 'considering a specialist assessment' and for 'suggestions for foster carers'.

Also includes a model for assessment, training tools, and forms for auditing social work practice and for reviewing multi-agency working.

NCB publications can be ordered from Central Books in any of the following ways:

Email: ncb@centralbooks.com Phone: 0845 458 9910 Post: download an order form and send it to National Children's Bureau, c/o Central Books, 99 Wallis Road, London E9 5LN Fax: you can fax your order form to Central Books on 0845 458 9912

Training and development resources

Crossing Bridges

Adrian Falkov, Kate Mayes and Marie Diggins

Published: 1999. Pavillion Publishing.

This publication provides comprehensive training for staff working with mentally ill parents and their children.

Commissioned by the Department of Health, this training resource has been designed to enhance practice and improve services for families in which mentally ill adults live together with dependent children. The training manual aims to improve individual practice whilst encouraging inter-agency collaboration across specialist areas. The key approach of the training works on the premise that children and their mentally ill parents are better supported and protected if agencies coordinate services and interventions.

http://www.pavpub.com/pavpub/trainingmaterials/showfull.asp?Section=1&Subsection=7&Product=178

Keeping the Family in Mind

The Keeping the Family in Mind project undertaken by Barnardo's has produced an information pack and a video made by young carers whose parents have experienced mental health problems. It is a useful resource for professionals, including adult mental health, and children and families professionals. For further details, contact:

Louise Wardale
Keeping the Family in Mind Coordinator
Barnardo's Action with Young Carers
24 Colquitt Street
Liverpool
L1 4DE
0151 708 7323

http://www.barnardos.org.uk/youngcarersnorthwest/young_carers_north_west_contact_us.htm

Being Seen and Heard

This training pack from the Royal College of Psychiatrists comprises a DVD/video with a CD-ROM of additional resources and a copy of The Royal College of Psychiatrists' report *Patients as Parents* (2002).

The training film has been developed for the use of staff involved in the care of mentally ill parents and their children – whether from the health, social care, education, probation or voluntary sector services.

Part I shows children and parents relating their various experiences of the referral process. Part II focuses on solutions and the ways in which professionals can help. The stories are interspersed with comments from experts.

The parents and children who have contributed to the film have given their permission on the strict understanding that the film will be used for training purposes only.

http://www.rcpsych.ac.uk/campaigns/partnersincare/beingseenandheard.aspx

Bibliography

Abdulrahim, D 'Black and Minority Ethnic Drug Use' in Hart, D and Powell, J (eds)(2006) *Adult Drug Problems, Children's Needs: Assessing the impact of parental drug use – A toolkit for practitioners.* National Children's Bureau.

ACMD (Advisory Council on the Misuse of Drugs) (2005) *Government Response to Hidden Harm: The report of an inquiry by the Advisory Council on the Misuse of Drugs.* Department for Education and Skills.

Aldridge, T (1999) 'Family Values: Rethinking children's needs living with drug abusing parents', *Druglink*, March/April, 8–11.

Aldridge, J and Becker, S (2003) *Children Who Care for Parents with Mental Illness: The perspectives of young carers, parents and professionals.* Policy Press.

Allport, G (1954) *The Nature of Prejudice.* New York: Addison-Wesley.

Bancroft, A and others (2004) *Parental Drug and Alcohol Misuse: Resilience and transition among young people.* Joseph Rowntree Foundation.

Barnard, MA and Barlow, J (2003) 'Discovering parental drug dependence: silence and disclosure', *Children and Society*, 17, 1, 45–56.

Bates, T and others (1999) *Drug Use, Parenting and Child Protection: Towards an effective interagency response.* University of Central Lancashire.

Bee, H (2000) *The Developing Child.* Needham Heights, MA: Allyn and Bacon.

Bennett, G (1989) *Treating Drug Abusers.* Routledge.

Bennet, L and others (1987) 'Couples at risk for alcoholism recurrence: Protective influences', *Family Process*, 26, 111–129.

Brisby, T, Baker, S and Hedderwick, T (1997) *Under the Influence: Coping with parents who drink too much. A report on the needs of children and problem drinking parents.* Alcohol Concern.

Brody, S (2006) 'Family placement: Special guardians – special report', *Community Care*, 6 October.

Cabinet Office, Social Exclusion Taskforce (2004) *Mental Health and Social Exclusion.* Cabinet Office.

Cabinet Office, Social Exclusion Taskforce (2007) *Reaching Out: Think family – Analysis and themes from the Families At Risk Review.* Cabinet Office.

Cabinet Office, Social Exclusion Taskforce (2008) *Think Family: Improving the life chances of families at risk.* Cabinet Office.

Cade, B and O'Hanlon, WH (1993) *A Brief Guide to Brief Therapy.* WW Norton.

Calder, Martin C and Hackett, S (eds) (2003) *Assessment in Childcare: Using and developing frameworks for practice.* Russell House Publishing.

ChildLine (1997) *Beyond the Limit: Children who live with parental alcohol misuse.* ChildLine.

Cleaver, H, Unell, I and Aldgate, J (1999) *Children's Needs, Parenting Capacity: The impact of parental mental illness, problem alcohol and drug use, and domestic violence on children's development.* Department of Health and The Stationery Office.

Commission for Social Care Inspection (2006) *Supporting Parents, Safeguarding Children: Meeting the needs of parents with children on the child protection register.* CSCI.

Corrigan, PW (ed) (2004) *On the Stigma of Mental Illness: Practical strategies for research and social change.* American Psychological Association.

Dalzell, R and Sawyer, E (2011) *Putting Analysis into Assessment: Undertaking assessments of need – A toolkit for practitioners.* Second edition. NCB.

Dearden, C and Becker, S (2004) *Young Carers in the UK: The 2004 report.* Carers National Association.

Department for Education and Skills (2005a) *Statutory Guidance on the Roles and Responsibilities of the Director of Children's Services and Lead Member for Children's Services.* DfES.

Department for Education and Skills (2005b) *Children's Workforce Strategy: A strategy to build a world-class workforce for children and young people consultation.*

Department for Education and Skills (2006a) *Parenting Support. Guidance for Local Authorities in England. October 2006.* Department for Education and Skills. *http://www.everychildmatters.gov.uk*

Department for Education and Skills (2006b) *Children's Services: The market for parental and family support services.* Department for Education and Skills.

Department for Education and Skills and Department of Health (2006) *Joint Planning and Commissioning Framework for Children, Young People and Maternity Services.* Department for Education and Skills. *www.everychildmatters.gov.uk/strategy/planningandcommissioning*

Department for Education (2011) *Family and Friends Care: Statutory Guidance for Local Authorities.*

Department of Health (1999) *National Service Framework for Mental Health: Modern standards and service models.* Department of Health.

Department of Health (2000) *Framework for the Assessment of Children in Need and their Families.* The Stationery Office.

Department of Health (2002) *Mental Health Policy Implementation Guide: Dual diagnosis good practice guide.* Department of Health.

Department of Health (2003a) *Fair Access to Care Services: Guidance on eligibility criteria for adult social care.* (LAC (2002)13). Department of Health.

Department of Health (2003b) *Delivering Race Equality: A framework for action.* Department of Health.

Department of Health (2004) *National Service Framework for Children, Young People and Maternity Services.* Department of Health.

Department of Health (2005) *Delivering Race Equality in Mental Health Care: An action plan for reform inside and outside services and the Government's response to the independent inquiry into the death of David Bennett.* Department of Health.

Department of Health (2006) *Guidance on the Statutory Chief Officer Post of the Director of Adult Social Services.* Department of Health.

Department of Health and Social Services Inspectorate (2000) *Modern Social Services: A commitment to people. The 9th annual report of the Chief Inspector of Social Services 1999/2000.* Department of Health.

Edwards, R and Gillies, V (2005) *Resources in Parenting: Access to Capitals Project Report.* University of South Bank. *Families & Social Capital.* ESRC Research Group.

Elliot, E and Watson, A (1998) *Fit To Be A Parent: The needs of drug using parents in Salford and Trafford.* Manchester Public Health and Research Centre, University of Salford.

Erikson, JR and Henderson, AD (1992) 'Witnessing family violence: The children's experience', *Journal of Advanced Nursing,* 17, 1200–1209.

Fahlberg, VMD (1991) *A Child's Journey Through Placement.* Perspectives Press.

Falkov, A (ed) (1998) *Crossing Bridges: Training resources for working with mentally ill parents and their children. Reader – for managers, practitioners and trainers.* Department of Health.

Family Rights Group (2008) *The role of the state in supporting relatives raising children who cannot live with their parents: A submission to the House of Commons' Children, Schools and Families Select Committee – Looked-after Children Enquiry by Family Rights Group* (March). http://www.frg. org.uk/policy_papers.html

Family Welfare Association (2008) *Families Affected by Parental Mental Health Difficulties.* Family Welfare Association.

Famularo, R, Kinscherff, R and Fenton, T (1992) 'Parental substance abuse and the nature of child maltreatment', *Child Abuse and Neglect,* 16, 4, 475–483.

Fonagy, P and others (1994) 'The theory and practice of resilience', *Journal of Child Psychology and Psychiatry,* 35, 2, 231–257.

Forrester, D (2000) 'Parental substance misuse and child protection in a British sample: A survey of children on the child protection register in an inner-London district office', *Child Abuse Review,* 9, 4, Jul/Aug, 235–246.

Forrester, D 'Social work assessments with parents who misuse drugs or alcohol' in Phillips, R (2004) *Children Exposed to Parental Substance Misuse: Implications for family placement.* BAAF.

Forrester, D and Harwin, J (2006) 'Parental substance misuse and child care social work: Findings from the first stage of a study of 100 families', *Child & Family Social Work,* 11, 4, Nov, 325–335.

Forrester, D and others (2008) 'How do child and family social workers talk to parents about child welfare concerns?' *Child Abuse Review,* 17, 1, Jan/Feb, 23–35.

FRANK – website *www.talktofrank.com*

Frank, J (1995) *Couldn't Care More: A study of young carers and their needs.* The Children's Society.

Fraser, C and others (2006) 'Interventions programmes for children of parents with a mental illness: A critical review', *International Journal of Mental Health Promotion,* 8, 1, Feb.

Fuller, R and others (2000) *Young People and Welfare: Negotiating pathways.* University of Stirling, ESRC.

Ghate, D, Shaw, C and Hazel, N (2000) *How Family Centres are Working with Fathers.* Joseph Rowntree Foundation.

Gopfert, M, Webster, J and Seeman, M (eds) (2004) *Parental Psychiatric Disorder: Distressed parents and their families.* Cambridge University Press.

Gorin, S (2004) *Understanding What Children Say: Children's experiences of domestic violence, parental substance misuse and parental health problems.* National Children's Bureau.

Greene, R, Pugh, R and Roberts, D (2008) *Black and Minority Ethnic Parents with Mental Health Problems and their Children.* Research Briefing, 29, SCIE (Social Care Institute for Excellence).

Grotberg, E (1995) *A Guide to Promoting Resilience in Children: Strengthening the human spirit.* The Hague, Holland: Bernard van Leer Foundation.

Gruer, L and Ainsworth, T (2003) *Hidden Harm: Responding to the needs of children of problem drug users. The report of an Inquiry by the Advisory Council on the Misuse of Drugs.* Home Office.

Hackett, S (eds) (2003) *Assessment in Childcare: Using and developing frameworks for practice.* Russell House Publishing.

Hamer, M (2005) *Preventing Breakdown: A manual for those working with families and the individuals within them.* Russell House Publishing.

Hamilton, C and Collins, J 'The role of alcohol in wife beating and child abuse: A review of the literature' in Collins, J (ed) (1981) *Drinking and Crime.* New York: Guilford Press.

Harbin, F and Murphy, M (eds) (2000) *Substance Misuse and Child Care: How to understand, assist and intervene when drugs affect parenting.* Russell House.

Hart, D and Powell, J (2006) *Adult Drug Problems, Children's Needs: Assessing the impact of parental drug use – A toolkit for practitioners*. National Children's Bureau.

Harwin and others (2011) *The Family Drug and Alcohol Court (FDAC) Evaluation Project Final Reports*. Brunel University.

Healthcare Commission (2005) *Count Me In: Results of a national census of inpatients in mental health hospitals and facilities in England and Wales*, Healthcare Commission.

Hester, M, Pearson, C and Harwin, N 'Making an impact: Children and domestic violence – a reader' in Kroll, B and Taylor, A (2003) *Parental Substance Misuse and Child Welfare*. Jessica Kingsley.

Hinshaw, S (2005) 'The stigmatization of mental illness in children and parents: Developmental issues, family concerns, and research needs', *Journal of Child Psychology and Psychiatry*, 46, 7, 714–734.

HM Government (2006a) *Working Together to Safeguard Children: A guide to inter-agency working to safeguard and promote the welfare of children*. HM Government.

HM Government (2006b) *Common Assessment Framework guides*. HM Government. *http://www.everychildmatters.gov.uk/resources-and-practice/IG00063/*

HM Government (2008) *Drugs: Protecting families and communities. The 2008 drug strategy*. HM Government.

Holland, S (2004*) Child and Family Assessment in Social Work Practice*. Sage.

Hollows, A 'Making professional judgements in the framework for the assessment of children in need and their families' in Calder, Martin C and Hackett, S (eds) (2003) *Assessment in Childcare: Using and developing frameworks for practice*. Russell House Publishing.

Home Office, Department of Health and Department for Education (1995) *Tackling Drugs Together: A strategy for England 1995–1998*. (Cm 2846). HMSO.

Jack, G (1997) 'An ecological approach to social work with children and families', *Child and Family Social Work*, 2, 109–120.

Jack, G and Gill, O (2003) *The Missing Side of the Triangle: Assessing the importance of family and environmental factors in the lives of children*. Barnardo's.

Jordan, L and Lindley, B (eds) (2006) *Special Guardianship: What does it offer children who cannot live with their parents?* Family Rights Group.

Kearney, P, Levin, E and Rosen, G (2003) *Alcohol, Drug and Mental Health Problems: Working with families* (SCIE Reports No.2). Social Care Institute for Excellence.

Kearney, P and others (2003) *Families That Have Alcohol and Mental Health Problems: A template for partnership working* (SCIE Resource Guides No.1). Social Care Institute for Excellence.

Kroll, B and Taylor, A (2003) *Parental Substance Misuse and Child Welfare*. Jessica Kingsley.

Kurtz, Z and others (2005) *Minority Voices: A guide to good practice in planning and providing services for the mental health of black and minority ethnic young people*. Young Minds.

Laybourn, A, Brown, J and Hill, M (1996) *Hurting on the Inside: Children's experience of parental alcohol misuse*. Avebury.

Leese, M and others (2006) 'Ethnic differences among patients in high-security psychiatric hospitals in England', *British Journal of Psychiatry*, 188: 380–385.

Link, BG and others (1997) 'On stigma and its consequences: Evidence from a longitudinal study of men with dual diagnoses of mental illness and substance abuse', *Journal of Health and Social Behaviour*, 38, 177–190.

Lyall, J (2006) 'The struggle for "cultural competence"', *Guardian*, 12 April.

McAleavy, S, Pearson, H and Sloan, H (2004) *Can You See The Elephant? A toolkit for talking to children and young people about parental substance use*. Leicestershire Partnership NHS Trust, Leicester City Council and DRUG Alcohol Response Team

McCracken, DG (1988) *The Long Interview.* Beverly Hills, CA: Sage.

Meltzer, H and others (1995) *The Prevalence of Psychiatric Morbidity among Adults Aged 16–64 Living in Private Households in Great Britain* (OPCS Surveys: Report 1). OPCS.

Melzer, D (2003) 'Inequalities in mental health: A "systematic review" in The Research Findings register', Summary no. 1063 in Family Welfare Association (2008) *Families Affected by Parental Mental Health Difficulties.* Family Welfare Association.

Miller, NS (ed) (1994) *Treating Coexisting Psychiatric and Addictive Disorders.* Hazelden: Minnesota.

Miller, WR and Rollnick, S (2002) *Motivational Interviewing: Preparing people for change.* Guilford Press.

Morris, J and Wates, M (2006) *Supporting Disabled Parents and Parents with Additional Support Needs.* Knowledge Review 11, Social Care Institute for Excellence (SCIE). http://www.scie.org.uk/publications/details.asp?pubID=107

Mullender, A and others (2002) *Children's Perspectives on Domestic Violence.* Sage.

NSPCC (2000) *The Child's World: Assessing children in need.* National Society for the Prevention of Cruelty to Children.

Newman, T and Blackburn, S (2002) *Transitions in the Lives of Children and Young People: Resilience factors* (Interchange 78). Scottish Executive.

Olsen, R and Wates, M (2003) *Disabled Parents: Examining research assumptions.* Dartington and Research in Practice.

Patel, N (ed) (2000) *Clinical Psychology, Race, and Culture: A training manual.* British Psychological Society.

Phillips, E (ed) (2004) *Children Exposed to Parental Substance Misuse: Implications for family placement.* BAAF.

Powers, R (1986) 'Aggression and violence in the family' in Campbell, A and Gibbs, J (1986) *Violent Transactions.* Blackwells.

Prime Minister's Strategy Unit (2003) *Alcohol Harm Reduction Project: Interim analytical report.* Cabinet Office. http://www.strategy.gov.uk/downloads/files/su%20interimreport2.pdf

Prochaska, JO, Norcross, JC and Diclemente, CC (1994) *Changing for Good: The revolutionary program that explains the six stages of change and teaches you how to free yourself from bad habits.* William Morrow & Co.

Roberts, AR (1990) *Crisis Intervention Handbook: Assessment, treatment and research.* Belmont CA: Wadsworth.

Rogers, Carl (1962) *On Becoming a Person: A therapist's view of psychotherapy.* Constable.

Royal College of Psychiatrists (2002) *Patients as Parents: Addressing the needs, including the safety of children whose parents have mental illness.* Royal College of Psychiatrists.

Royal College of Psychiatrists (2008) *Parental Mental Illness: The problems for children, for parents and teachers* (Factsheet 16). Royal College of Psychiatrists.

Rutter, M (1993) 'Resilience: Some conceptual considerations', *Journal of Adolescent Health,* 14, 626–631.

Rutter, M (1999) 'Resilience concepts and findings: Implications for family therapy', *Journal of Family Therapy,* 21, 119–144.

Ryan, M (2000) *Working with Fathers.* Radcliffe Medical Press.

The Sainsbury Centre for Mental Health (2006) *The Costs of Race Inequality (Policy Paper 6).* London: The Sainsbury Centre for Mental Health. http://www.scmh.org.uk/publications/costs_of_race_inequality.aspx?ID=504

Sartorius, N (1998) 'Stigma: What can psychiatrists do about it? *Lancet,* 352, 1058–1059.

Scott, D (1998) 'A qualitative study of social work assessment in cases of alleged child abuse', *British Journal of Social Work,* 28, 1, 73–88.

Shaw, C (2005a) *Evaluation Toolkit: A tailored approach to evaluation for parenting projects.* Parenting Education and Support Forum, and National Children's Bureau.

Shaw, C (2005b) *NIFTY Evaluation: An introductory handbook for social care staff with a rough guide to evaluation resources.* Research in Practice in partnership with NCB.

Sheldon, B 'The psychology of incompetence', in Blom-Cooper, L (ed) (1987) *After Beckford: Essays on themes connected with the case of Jasmine Beckford.* London. Royal Holloway and Bedford New College.

Singleton, N and others, '*Psychiatric morbidity among adults living in private households'*, in Social Exclusion Unit (2004) *Mental Health and Social Exclusion.* Office of the Deputy Prime Minister.

Social Exclusion Unit (2004) *Mental Health and Social Exclusion.* Office of the Deputy Prime Minister. http://www.socialinclusion.org.uk/publications/SEU.pdf

Thornicroft, G (2006) *Actions Speak Louder… Tackling discrimination against people with mental illness.* Mental Health Foundation.

Treasure, J (2004) 'Motivational interviewing', *Advances in Psychiatric Treatment,* 10, 331–337.

Tunnard, J (2002a) *Parental Drug Misuse: A review of impact and intervention studies.* Research in Practice.

Tunnard, J (2002b) *Parental Problem Drinking and its Impact on Children.* Research in Practice.

Tunnard, J (2004) *Parental Mental Health Problems: Messages from research, policy and practice.* Research in Practice.

Turnell, A and Edwards, S (1999) *Signs of Safety: A solution and safety-orientated approach to child protection.* WW Norton and Co.

Turning Point (2006) *Bottling it up: The effects of alcohol misuse on children, parents and families.* Turning Point.

Velleman, R (1993) *Alcohol and the Family.* Institute of Alcohol Studies.

Velleman, R 'Alcohol and drug problems in parents: An overview of the impact on children and implications for practice' in Gopfert, M, Webster, J and Seeman, M (2004) (eds) *Parental Psychiatric Disorder: Distressed parents and their families.* Cambridge University Press.

Velleman, R and Orford, J (1993) 'The importance of family discord in explaining childhood problems', *Addiction Research,* 1, 1, 36–57.

Velleman, R and Orford, J (1999) *Risk and Resilience: Adults who were the children of problem drinkers.* Harwood.

Wahl, OF (1995) *Media Madness: Public images of mental illness.* New Brunswick, New Jersey: Rutgers University Press.

Wates, M (2002) *Supporting Disabled Adults in their Parenting Role.* Joseph Rowntree Foundation. York Publishing Service.

Weissman, MM and Paykel, ES (1974) *The Depressed Woman: A study of social relationships.* Chicago: University of Chicago Press.

World Health Organisation (1992) *The ICD10 Classification of Mental and Behavioural Disorders: Clinical Descriptions and Diagnostic Guidelines.* Geneva. WHO.

Appendix 1: Agencies who participated in the Building Resilience project

1. Borough of Telford and Wrekin Children and Families Social Services (FAST)

2. Bracknell Forest Borough Council, Children's Services

3. Child and Adolescent Mental Health Services, North Essex Mental Health Partnerships NHS Trust

4. SureStart High Cross, Haringey

5. NSPCC Family Alcohol Service and Parkside

6. Greenwich Social Services Children and Family/Mental Health Project – CAPE

7. CAN, Northampton

8. Core Kids, London

9. Birmingham and Solihull Substance Misuse Service, Birmingham and Solihull Mental Health NHS Trust

10. Suffolk Family Group Conferencing Service, Suffolk County Council

11. ADAS (Alcohol and Drugs Advisory Service), Harlow, Essex

12. BADAS (Barnsley Alcohol and Drugs Advisory Service), Barnsley

13. Brighton Oasis Project, Brighton

14. Children and Families Division, Southampton City Council

15. ARCH Initiatives (Substance Misuse Services), Wirral

16. Southend-on-Sea Primary Care Trust with Southend MIND

17. Family Support and Child Protection Team, Lambeth Social Services with Lambeth CAMHS

18. The Meriden West Midlands Family Programme

19. Co-ordinator, Children in Families with Mental Illness and CAMHS, London Borough of Tower Hamlets and East London and City Mental Health Trust

20. East City Community Mental Health Team, Oxfordshire

21. Newham Asian Women's Project, Plaistow

22. Parental Substance Misuse Service, Greenwich

23. Bristol Children and Young People's Service

Appendix 2: Legislation and policy context

This appendix covers the following relevant areas of policy and law.

1. Cross-cutting policy and legislation

2. Children's and adult social care

3. Health and social care reform

4. Welfare reform

5. Community care

6. Mental health

7. Drugs and alcohol

8. Families and parenting

9. Young carers

10. Disability

1. Cross-cutting policy and legislation

Human Rights Act 1998

The government incorporated the European Convention on Human Rights into UK law in 1998, creating the Human Rights Act. The most relevant articles are:

- Article 3, which prohibits inhuman and degrading treatment
- Article 8, which guarantees the right to respect for private and family life
- Article 14, prohibiting discrimination in the enjoyment of Convention rights.

Article 8 is of particular significance, since it prohibits any arbitrary interference with the right to a private and family life. For example, case law stipulates that, even though a child may be taken into care for his or her protection, that does not allow for the relationship between the child and birth parent to be terminated unless this is in the best interests of the child.

Article 3 stipulates that protection rights are absolute, so children should be protected from all forms of inhuman and degrading treatment. What is less clear, however, is the demarcation line under article 3 that requires that action be taken by social services or other state agencies to protect that child.

UN Convention on the Rights of the Child (CRC)

The UK government ratified the CRC in 1991, while it formerly reserved the right to insist as the privacy of UK immigration law over Convention rights, this reservation was withdrawn in 2008. The CRC has not been incorporated into UK law and, unlike the European Convention of Human Rights, has no court system attached to ensure that it is understood and implemented.

The most relevant articles are:

- **Article 3** – best interests of the child (in all actions, the best interests of the child shall be a primary consideration)
- **Article 5** – parental guidance (which deals with the responsibilities, rights and duties of parents for their child)
- **Article 9** – separation from parents (which ensures that a child may not be separated from his or her parents against their will, unless it is necessary to protect the child from harm, or in cases involving parental separation that specify a child's place of residence)
- **Article 19** – protection from abuse and neglect.

Equality Act 2010

The Equality Act 2010 aims to consolidate all previous anti-discrimination and equality legislation, as well as strengthening protection from discrimination, harassment or victimisation in relation to age, disability, gender, race, religion or belief, sexuality, gender reassignment, marriage and civil partnership and pregnancy and maternity. It also introduces a new 'public sector equality duty', requiring all public agencies to eliminate unlawful discrimination, harassment or victimisation, and to promote equality of opportunity and good relations. In addition, certain public bodies (including government departments, local authorities and the NHS) are given a duty to consider how their decisions might help to reduce socio-economic inequalities. Measures in the Equality Act 2006 that established the Equality and Human Rights Commission (EHRC), to enforce anti-discriminatory legislation and promote a culture of respect for human rights, remain in force.

Children's services

The Children Act 2004 provides the legislative framework for the previous government's Every Child Matters agenda, which sought to strengthen partnership working across agencies to promote children's well-being. While the current government has removed requirements to establish a Children's Trust Board and prepare a local authority Children and Young People's Plan, many of the original provisions of the 2004 Act remain in place:

- a reciprocal duty on a list of local partners (including local authorities, health services, the police and probation, schools and colleges and youth offending teams) to cooperate to improve the well-being of children (section 10)

- a definition of child well-being: physical and mental health and emotional well-being; protection from harm and neglect; access to education, training and recreation; making a contribution to society; and social and economic well-being (section 10)

- a duty on partners to safeguard and promote the welfare of children (section 11)

- every local authority having to appoint a Director of Children's Services and a named councillor (lead member) with responsibility for children's services (sections 18 and 19)

- the requirement that each local area have a Local Safeguarding Children Board (section 13)

The Act did not legislate for key elements of the Every Child Matters agenda, including: the Common Assessment Framework (a standardised initial assessment form for all staff), the Lead Professional (a named individual who acts as a single point of contact for children who require a package of service provision), and the Team Around the Child (TAC) (a multi-disciplinary team of practitioners established on a case-by-case basis to support a child, young person or family). However, the current government continues to promote these approaches. On the other hand, work to implement ContactPoint – a database to help practitioners working with children share information and legislated for in this Act – was ceased by the current government.

Cross-government guidance on the Children Act 2004 and partnership working

Placing an emphasis on cutting bureaucracy and local discretion, the coalition government has reduced the quantity of guidance relating to Children Act 2004 measures. Government guidance currently comprises:

- *Information Sharing: Guidance for practitioners and managers* (HM Government 2008)
- *Working Together to Safeguard Children: A guide to inter-agency working to safeguard and promote the welfare of children* (includes guidance on Local Safeguarding Children Boards) (HM Government 2010)
- *The Framework for Assessment of Children in Need and their Families* (Department of Health and others 2000)
- Information on the Common Assessment Framework (CAF) processes and practical tools for using the framework http://www.education.gov.uk/childrenandyoungpeople/strategy/ integratedworking/a0068944/team-around-the-child-tac

The government also endorses and promotes the Children's Workforce Development Council guidance, *Team Around the Child and the lead professional: guides for managers and practitioners* (Children's Workforce Development Council 2009). (See http://www.education. gov.uk/childrenandyoungpeople/strategy/integratedworking/a0068961/the-lead-professional, last accessed December 2011). Statutory guidance on Children's Trusts was withdrawn by the coalition government in Autumn 2010, reflecting the Department for Education's emphasis on giving local areas discretion around their partnership and planning arrangements.

Children's services inspection arrangements

While the Children Act 2004 set out arrangements for joint inspections of children's services, which became part of the Comprehensive Area Assessment in 2009, inspection arrangements are currently subject to change. The new coalition government abolished the Comprehensive Area Assessment when it came into power. In July 2011, Ofsted carried out a public consultation on proposals for local authority children's services inspections to focus on the effectiveness of local authority and partners' services for children who may be at risk of harm, including the effectiveness of early identification and early help, and on services for children in care. New arrangements will come into force in May 2012.

2. Children's and adult social care

Children Act 1989

The Children Act 1989 is the major child-centred piece of social welfare legislation. Section 1 contains the heart of the Act: the welfare of the child should be the core consideration whenever a court is required to make a decision regarding the upbringing of a child, or administration of a child's property. The Act introduces the concept of parental responsibility – given automatically to birth mothers and married fathers, and upon application to an unmarried father – which in law refers to 'the rights, duties, powers, responsibilities and authority which by law a parent of a child has in relation to the child and his property'.

Parents who separate may still have parental responsibility and are expected to maintain some involvement in their child's life.

When considering the welfare of a child, the court uses the welfare checklist as a framework within which to make its decision. The checklist comprises:

- the ascertainable wishes and feelings of the child concerned (considered in the light of his age and understanding)
- his physical, emotional and educational needs
- the likely effect on him of any change in his circumstances
- his age, sex, background and any characteristics of his which the court considers relevant
- any harm which he has suffered or is at risk of suffering
- how capable each of his parents, and any other person in relation to whom the court considers the question to be relevant, is of meeting his needs
- the range of powers available to the court.

Part III of the Act deals with local authority duties. Section 17 deals with the provision of services for children in need. A child is 'in need' if: he or she is unlikely to achieve or maintain, or to have the opportunity of achieving or maintaining, a reasonable standard of health or development without the provision of services; or, the child's health or development is likely to be significantly impaired, or further impaired, without the provision of such services; or the child is disabled.

Children who are suffering or at risk of suffering 'significant harm' may be taken into the care of the local authority. The harm must be attributable to the care given to the child, or the child being beyond parental control.

Munro review of child protection

In June 2010, the coalition government commissioned Professor Eileen Munro to conduct a review of the child protection system. Her final report (Department for Education 2011a) was published in May 2011, followed by government's response in July of the same year (Department for Education 2011b). Munro emphasised the need to 'move from a compliance to a learning culture', allowing freedom for social workers to use their professional judgement. Her recommendations included measures to: remove unhelpful targets, IT systems and guidelines; secure early help for families who do not meet the criteria for social care services to prevent problems escalating; and keep experienced social workers on the front line. In response government has committed to:

- revise *Working Together to Safeguard Children* statutory guidance by July 2012 with earlier interim amendments

- publish a suite of new nationally collected performance data on child protection services by May 2012
- consider how to ensure local authorities and their partners secure provision of early help (including whether a statutory duty would be appropriate)
- work with local authorities to review and redesign the ways in which child and family social work is delivered, drawing on evidence of what works
- encourage all local authorities to designate a Principal Child and Family Social Worker
- develop a joint Department for Education and Department for Health work programme to promote improved safeguarding practice in the context of the health reforms (published October 2011, see http://www.education.gov.uk/munroreview/downloads/ DHDfEJointWorkProgramme2.pdf, last accessed December 2011).

Adult social care

In November 2010, the government published its vision for adult social care, including an emphasis on partnership working as a means of identifying wider individual and family needs and safeguarding children (Department of Health, 2010a). The 2011/12 adult social care outcomes framework, however, includes no focus on children dependent on adults in receipt of social services. In late 2011, the government carried out a consultation process, gathering views on the future of adult social care, including exploring how services can support better prevention and early intervention and be more integrated. A white paper is expected in spring 2012.

Two pieces of government guidance on the role of the Director of Adult Services – statutory and best practice - look at the links that should be made between adult and children's social services and, in particular, the complementary roles of the Director of Adult Social Services (DASS) and the Director of Children's Services (DCS) (Department of Health 2006a, Department of Health 2006b). The DASS is responsible for the local needs assessment, the planning and commissioning of services, workforce planning and managing cultural change, driving partnership working, promoting social inclusion and well-being, and delivering an integrated approach to supporting the adult community. The needs of families are recognised, and the best practice guidance recommends establishing clear protocols between adult and children's services, and making sure that procedures for joint working are in place to ensure that the needs of, or risk to, the child are considered when a social worker is assessing the needs of or providing a service to the parent.

Guidance on eligibility criteria for adult social care in England states that, in the course of assessing an individual's needs, local authorities should: recognise that adults with dependent children may require help with their parenting responsibilities; and ensure that children are not expected to take on inappropriate levels of caring responsibilities (Department of Health 2010b). (See below for more on Young Carers.)

3. Health and social care reform

The coalition government is implementing wide-ranging reform to the commissioning and delivery of NHS, public health and social care services, a key aim of which is the better integration of health and social care services (Department of Health 2010c, Department of Health 2010d). Subject to approval by parliament, The Health and Social Care bill will abolish Primary Care Trusts, transferring responsibility for commissioning most NHS services to new GP-led clinical commissioning groups (CCGs). Local authorities will take on the majority of public health commissioning. At the national level, the new NHS Commissioning Board will oversee NHS commissioning and commission some specialist health services (such as care for rare conditions or for the prison population), and NICE will develop quality standards for health and social care services.

To aid local integrated and partnership working, every local area will be required to have a Health and Well-being Board (HWB) to carry out the Joint Strategic Needs Assessment, and prepare a local joint health and well-being strategy. The HWB will bring together local CCGs, the Directors of Adult and Children's Services and the Director of Public Health – providing a forum through which decisions may be taken on the needs of vulnerable families.

The National Service Framework for Children, Young People and Maternity Services (Department of Health/Department for Education and Skills 2004) was the previous government's ten-year plan for improving health services for children and families. The framework has been less prominent in the context of the current government's reforms to the health service. In the future, progress in improving services will be measured through the NHS, public health and adult social care outcomes frameworks.

4. Welfare reform

The government is introducing a programme of changes to the welfare system, through its welfare reform white paper (Department for Work and Pensions 2010) and the Welfare Reform Bill [going through Parliament at the time of writing]. Existing work-related benefits – including Income Support (for those on low incomes), Employment and Support Allowance (for those who are unable to work because of illness or disability), Jobseeker's Allowance, Housing Benefit, Child Tax Credit and Working Tax Credit – will be integrated into a single Universal Credit (UC). The single basic UC payment, providing for basic living costs, will be augmented by additional amounts for certain circumstances, including: disability; caring responsibilities; housing costs; number of children; and childcare. There will be a phased approach to the introduction of Universal Credit starting in 2013, and it is expected to take ten years to come fully into effect.

The government's 2010 Spending Review (HM Treasury 2010) announced a cap on household benefit, although those receiving Disability Living Allowance, War Widows and working families will be exempt from this cap. Some recipients will face an increasing level of conditionality, which will come into force ahead of the introduction of the Universal Credit. Recipients of Income Support, Employment and Support Allowance or Jobseeker's Allowance will be subject to a 'claimant commitment', outlining the requirements expected of benefit recipients, with tougher sanctions if these are not met.

5. Community care

NHS and Community Care Act 1990

This introduced the term 'care management' – separating the roles of assessment and care planning with service provision. Disabled people (see definitions in Disability section at the end of this document) are entitled to assessments for services. Seven stages of care management are set out in the guidance: publishing information, determining the level of assessment, assessing need, care planning, implementing the care plan, monitoring, and reviewing.

The Care Programme Approach (CPA)

Introduced in 1991, implementation of this approach for services for people with mental illness was led by health authorities and involves individual packages of care for all patients prior to discharge and for those using specialist psychiatric services.

Key elements include: an assessment of need, care planning, allocation of a key worker, and regular reviews of progress. A tiered care programme has been developed, with a full multidisciplinary CPA for those with severe and enduring mental health problems; and those assessed as having less complex needs receiving a less intensive form of CPA. All agencies should agree a single care plan, have a single key worker and everyone should know who that is.

There is local discretion as to how to implement this, so there is considerable local variation.

6. Mental health

Mental Health Act 1983 and the Code of Practice

The Mental Health Act 1983 – amended by the Mental Health Act 2007 – provides a framework for compulsory admissions to hospital, treatment in the community, and provisions for the care of in-patients and aftercare. It sets out the following broad principles: respect and consideration of individual qualities; needs taken fully into account; treatment or care to be in the least controlled and segregated facilities practicable; and self-determination of service users to be supported as far as possible. Discharge from orders are to take place as soon as appropriate. The following are key sections.

- Section 2 – Compulsory admission for assessment (up to 28 days).
- Section 3 – Compulsory admission for treatment (up to 6 months renewable for a further 6 months, then annually).
- Section 4 – Compulsory admission in an emergency (where there is an urgent need for admission for assessment, and compliance with procedure under section 2 could cause undesirable delay). This lasts up to 72 hours and is for use in genuine emergencies. This is closely regulated by the Mental Health Act Commission and includes holding powers for doctors and nurses – Section 5(2) and 5(4).
- Section 37 – A hospital order can be made where someone is convicted of an offence who would normally receive a prison sentence.
- Section 117 – Aftercare: a duty on local authorities in relation to people who have been admitted under sections 3, 37, 45(a), 47 or 48 of the Act to provide aftercare on discharge.
- Section 136 – Police powers: where police can remove someone to a place of safety for up to 72 hours, the aim being to secure competent and speedy assessment by a doctor and Approved Social Worker (ASW) of the person. Local areas should have clear policies regarding the use of this.

Amendments introduced in the 2007 Act mean the following.

- The definition of 'mental disorder' has been broadened to mean 'any disorder or disability of the mind', although a safeguard has been added to ensure that a person with a learning disability may not be considered to be suffering from a mental disorder unless that disability is associated with abnormally aggressive or seriously irresponsible conduct on his part.
- The concept of 'treatability' has been replaced by an 'appropriate treatment' test, the effect of which will be that a detention may not take place unless appropriate medical treatment is available to the patient.

- The Approved Social Worker (ASW) has been replaced by the Approved Mental Health Professional (AMHP).
- Supervised community treatment for patients following a period in hospital has been introduced. Patients who fail to continue to receive their treatment may be made subject to a community treatment order, which places a number of conditions on a patient. These may include requirements regarding place of residence, availability at particular times and places for the purposes of medical treatment and/or examination, and a condition that the patient abstains from particular conduct.

An updated statutory Code of Practice contains a number of practice directions that relate to patients with mental health problems who are also parents (Department of Health 2008).

Mental health practice and policy documents

The coalition government's mental health strategy (HM Government 2011a) sets out priorities for promoting good mental health among all age groups. It highlights the importance of intervening early to address mental health problems, and in particular the damaging effect of a parent's poor mental health on their children. There is also an emphasis on: promoting 'positive parenting' as a means of preventing mental health problems among children and young people; parental anxiety and depression in the post-natal period and early years; and the importance of addressing the needs of children of a parent with mental health problems to prevent them from taking on inappropriate caring roles. Cross-government activity is set out under six objectives:

- more people of all ages and backgrounds will have better well-being and good mental health, with fewer people developing mental health problems
- more people who develop mental health problems will have a good quality of life, including a greater ability to manage their own lives, stronger social relationships and the skills they need for living and working and a suitable and stable place to live
- more people with mental health problems will have good physical health
- more people will have a positive experience of care and support, giving people the greatest choice and control over their own lives, in the least restrictive environment
- fewer people will suffer avoidable harm
- fewer people will experience stigma and discrimination.

Actions include: reforming Children's Centres to focus on the most disadvantaged families; £400 million over four years to give individuals a choice of psychological therapies to extend provision for people with severe mental illness and children and young people (among others); extending access to personal mental health budgets; and developing a long-term conditions (LTC) strategy for those with severe mental health conditions and those with an LTC also suffering from depression or anxiety. The government has also published a draft National Suicide Prevention Strategy for consultation (http://www.dh.gov.uk/en/Consultations/Liveconsultations/DH_128065, last accessed December 2011), and a final strategy will be published in 2012.

The *National Service Framework for Mental Health* (Department of Health, 1999) says little about parenting but does state the need for adult mental health professionals to be familiar with child protection procedures and acknowledges that it shouldn't be assumed that a child can provide the necessary caring responsibilities for their parent. It reinforces the need for more integrated working, strategic planning and commissioning and user involvement. It is supported by:

- Department of Health (2001) *The Mental Health Policy Implementation Guide.*
- Department of Health (2002) *Mental Health Policy Implementation Guide: Dual diagnosis good practice guide.*
- Department of Health (2002) *Women's Mental Health Strategy for England.*

Among the themes and action plans arising from the above is the SHIFT programme to tackle stigma and discrimination; and action plans to develop targeted support for parents with mental health problems and their families.

Social Care Institute for Excellence parental mental health and dual diagnosis resources

The Social Care Institute for Excellence (SCIE) has developed a range of resources on parental mental health and child welfare (including dual diagnosis), and provides good practice examples. (See http://www.scie.org.uk/topic/people/peoplewithmentalhealthproblems/ familieschildrenwhohavementalhealthproblems, last accessed December 2011).

7. Drugs and alcohol

Drug Strategy 2010

In December 2010, the coalition government published a revised drug strategy (HM Government 2010a). It addresses drug and alcohol dependency and highlights the association between mental illness and drug and alcohol dependence. There is an emphasis on preventing problems from arising, referring to government policies relating to Sure Start Children's Centres and interventions for families with multiple problems. Stating that children are sometimes 'invisible' to drug and alcohol services working with parents, the strategy stresses that children and adult services should work together to protect children, in accordance with *Working Together* statutory guidance, and encourages those working with children and families affected by substance misuse to undertake appropriate training. It encourages drug and alcohol, family and children's services to develop protocols for working together to respond to safeguarding concerns and support parents through treatment and in caring for their children, referring to National Treatment Agency guidelines (NTA 2011). The strategy states that drug and alcohol services should be represented on Local Safeguarding Children Boards.

While the drug strategy applies in part to government's approach to addressing alcohol misuse, the government has committed to publishing an Alcohol Strategy in early 2012.

Hidden Harm

In 2003, the Advisory Council on the Misuse of Drugs published research and policy recommendations on responding to the needs of children of problem drug users (Gruer and Ainsworth 2003). Their report, *Hidden Harm*, estimated that there were between 250,000 and 350,000 children of problem drug users in the UK. It notes that parental drug use can and does cause serious harm to children at every stage from conception to adulthood, and recommends that reducing the harm to children from parental problem drug use should become a main objective of policy and practice. The principle of services working together is highlighted, as is the recognition that effective treatment of the parent can have major benefits for the child.

Misuse of Drugs Act 1971

This Act categorises controlled drugs into three classes; with Class A drugs (that is, heroin, cocaine, ecstasy) considered to be the most harmful, and Class C drugs less harmful. For Class A drugs, the maximum sentence for possession is currently 7 years imprisonment and an unlimited fine; for supply, it is life imprisonment and an unlimited fine. The possession of Class B drugs can lead to a maximum 5 years imprisonment or a fine or both; and for supply, 14 years imprisonment or a fine or both. Drugs not covered by the Act include alcohol and solvents. However, the 1971 Act has been recently amended, giving the government powers to introduce 'temporary class drug orders' to tackle manufacturers of 'legal highs' (amended by the Police Reform and Social Responsibility Act 2011).

Criminal Justice Act 2003

Drug rehabilitation requirements

Drug testing and treatment orders were introduced in the Crime and Disorder Act 1998; and were replaced through the Criminal Justice Act 2003 by drug rehabilitation requirements in 2005. These are community orders which may be imposed on drug-dependent offenders who may be susceptible to treatment in areas where the appropriate services are deemed to be available. The order can last from between six months to three years, and can be applied only with the offender's consent subject to Parliamentary approval of the Legal Aid, Sentencing and Punishment of Offeders (LASPO) Bill, the requirement for a six month minimum period will be removed. If the offender refuses to comply with the order however, he can be subject to either a maximum £5,000 fine or a custodial sentence. The treatment provider – with treatment being either residential or non-residential – will act as the main supervisor of drug testing and the court may undertake periodic reviews, which must initially at least be attended by the offender.

Alcohol treatment requirement

The Criminal Justice Act 2003 also introduced an alcohol treatment requirement (ATR) that requires offenders to submit to a treatment for a period specified in the order, but of at least six months duration (six month minimum to be removed subject to Parliamentary approval of the LASPO Bill). The offender must consent to the giving of the ATR.

Drugs Act 2005

This Act updated previous drugs laws and introduced a number of new powers, including a power to test offenders for drug use on arrest rather than on charge. Those who test positive are required to undergo an assessment by a drugs worker.

Models of care for alcohol and drug misusers

In 2006, the Department of Health and NTA published a guide to the commissioning of alcohol services, including a short chapter on assessment that covers parenting responsibilities, and refers concerned professionals to the Local Safeguarding Children Board and social services. (NTA/Department of Health, 2006). A similar document provides national guidance on the commissioning and provision of treatment for adult drug misusers (NTA/Department of Health/ Home Office 2006). It sets out care pathways for parents or pregnant women known to be misusing drugs, and advocates a harm reduction approach with service users' children and families.

Other useful resources

Department of Health (England), the Scottish Government, Welsh Assembly Government and Northern Ireland Executive (2007) *Drug Misuse and Dependence: UK guidelines on clinical management.* London: The Stationery Office http://www.dh.gov.uk/en/ Publicationsandstatistics/Publications/PublicationsPolicyAndGuidance/DH_104819

The Social Care Institute for Excellence (SCIE) has developed a range of resources on substance misuse and dual diagnosis including *Families that have Alcohol and Mental Health Problems: A template for partnership working* (2003); and Working with families with alcohol, drug and mental health problems (2003)

http://www.scie.org.uk/topic/people/peoplewithmentalhealthproblems/ familieschildrenwhohavementalhealthproblems

Department of Health (2002) *Mental Health Policy Implementation Guide: Dual diagnosis good practice guide.*

8. Families and parenting

Early years

Supporting families in the foundation years (Department for Education/Department of Health 2011) brings together the government's policies around pregnancy to age five, and describes the systems needed to make the government's vision for services for children, parents and families of this age group a reality. It sits alongside a new website that provides advice and information to parents (see http://www.foundationyears.org.uk, last accessed December 2011). The document emphasises the importance of parental health and well-being to children's development, highlighting issues such as mental health, drug and alcohol misuse and poor family relationships. Actions government is taking to improve support for families in the early years include:

- encouraging greater provision and uptake of evidence-based parenting and relationship programmes, and training for Children's Centre staff to help them recognise and respond to families experiencing relationship difficulties
- doubling the number of families accessing the Family Nurse Partnership programme – a preventive programme, developed in the USA, providing intensive structured home visiting for young first time mothers
- recruiting a further 4,200 health visitors by 2015.
- trials of free parenting classes for mothers and fathers of children aged up to five in three local areas, for 50,000 parents, to stimulate a market in universal parenting classes by encouraging demand and supply.

Early intervention

In June 2010, the coalition government commissioned Graham Allen MP to conduct a review into early intervention, including how to secure, deliver and fund effective prevention and early intervention services (HM Government 2011b). The government's response to Allen's review has centred around its policies for the early years (described above). In addition, in the 2010 Spending Review, the government announced that local areas would receive an Early Intervention Grant (EIG), bringing together a range of funding streams for children, young people and families, including funding for family support, early years and youth services. While the EIG represents a cut in funding for these services and is not ring-fenced, the government is encouraging local areas to use this funding to support a range of services, including targeted support for families with multiple problems and ensuring Children's Centres are accessible to all but focusing support on the most vulnerable families.

Families with multiple problems

In December 2010, the prime minister set out an ambition to ensure that 120,000 families with multiple problems are helped to address their difficulties. Alongside the Early Intervention Grant (non ring-fenced funding for local authorities to spend on early intervention services needed in their local area), the prime minister announced that local areas would be able to pool funding for interventions for these families through 'community budgets', and that Government would provide funding to trial new approaches. Following the 'riots' in August 2011, the prime minister pledged to speed up this programme of work, and appointed Louise Casey to lead a troubled families team at the Department for Communities and Local Government.

Family and Friends Care

In 2011, the government issued long-awaited guidance to local authorities on family and friends care (DfE 2011d). This statutory guidance aims to improve outcomes for children and young people who, because they are unable to live with their parents, are being brought up by members of their extended families, friends or other people who are connected with them. In particular it provides guidance on the implementation of the duties in the Children Act 1989 in respect of such children and young people.

Anti-social behaviour

The previous government's programme to tackle anti-social behaviour had a significant focus on parenting. The Crime and Disorder Act 1998 introduced the Anti-Social Behaviour Order (ASBO) and the Parenting Order, since augmented by a number of interventions intended to compel parents to take responsibility for their child's problematic behaviour, whether in a criminal justice, housing or classroom context. The current coalition government carried out a consultation on anti-social behaviour reforms, proposing to abolish ASBOs and other court orders, replacing them with new measures that aim to restrict the behaviour of those who committed anti-social behaviour while also addressing underlying problems (which could include alcohol or substance misuse, or mental health problems). The government is yet to publicise its final plans, so details of how the current orders address parenting are set out below.

- **ASBOs** can be served against any person over the age of 10 years old. They have a minimum duration of two years and no statutory maximum duration – and can be imposed indefinitely at the discretion of the court. Although an ASBO is a civil remedy, breach of any of the conditions of an Order is a criminal offence, liable, in the case of an adult, to a maximum custodial sentence of 5 years and, in the case of a juvenile, to a maximum 24-month Detention and Training Order (DTO). (A DTO is the main custodial sentence for young people served half in custody and half in the community.) When children under 16 are given an ASBO, the court must consider whether it is appropriate to make a Parenting Order as well. Guidance for Youth Offending Teams in dealing with anti-social behaviour (Home Office/Youth Justice Board 2005) is currently being revised.
- **Acceptable Behaviour Contracts** are 'voluntary' and non-statutory. They often involve social housing landlords, the child, and his or her family. The contract refers to the need for the child to stop specific behaviours, and fulfil certain requirements like attending school regularly. It can also provide a list of what other public agencies should be offering the family in order to support this change in behaviour (for example, social services or education welfare). It should clarify what the repercussions would be if the terms of the contract are broken (and a repercussion could include being considered for an ASBO). What is less clear is any ramification if the public agency that should be providing a service fails to do so.
- **Individual Support Orders (ISOs)** were introduced in the Criminal Justice Act 2003. Magistrates' courts are obliged to make an ISO, when making an ASBO, if the court takes the view that it would prevent further anti-social behaviour. ISOs are intended to add to the ASBO by providing a list of 'positive conditions' based on an assessment of the child's needs that are intended to address the underlying causes of the anti-social behaviour. Youth Offending Teams coordinate ISO work with the child.
- **Parenting Orders** are court orders that require the named parents/carers to attend a parenting programme for up to three months. They can also place requirements on parents to deal with their child's behavioural issues. A breach of this can lead to a fine. **Parenting Contracts** are also 'voluntary' and non-statutory. However, a parent's refusal to agree to one, or failure to abide by its terms, can be cited in court as a reason to make a statutory Parenting Order. Guidance on Parenting Orders and contracts for Youth Offending Teams, the courts and other services was published in 2007 (Ministry of Justice/Youth Justice Board 2007).

Each of these interventions is intended to change the behaviour of the child, although good practice would also mean that any assessment of the parent's ability to parent could identify parental drug, alcohol or mental health problems. The multi-agency YOT would be able to refer any relevant case to its drug worker or health lead to ensure that a full assessment of the parent's needs could lead to an appropriate intervention.

School absence or truancy

The Education Act 1996 and Anti-Social Behaviour Act 2003 makes it clear that parents are obliged to ensure that their school-age children attend school regularly. If they fail to do so, they may be subject to a number of different interventions that can range from an informal interview with the head teacher, through to a more formal interview with an education welfare officer, and on to more punitive measures including Parenting Contracts, Parenting Orders, fines, or a community or custodial sentence. Guidance on education-related parenting contracts, parenting orders and penalty notices was published in 2007 (Department for Children, Schools and Families 2007).

9. Young carers

The coalition government published its strategy for carers in November 2010 (HM Government 2010b). Acknowledging that, in many cases, children of care users continue to be invisible to adult services, one of the key goals of the strategy is too ensure children and young people are protected from inappropriate caring and able to learn, develop and thrive. The strategy includes £400 million to provide carers, including young carers, with breaks from their caring responsibilities over the next four years. Support for young carers is another area of provision that local authorities are expected to fund through the Early Intervention Grant.

The carers strategy encourages a 'whole family' approach to assessing adults with caring requirements, so that both the service user and the carer can identify their own needs and to minimise the risk of young carers taking on inappropriate levels of responsibility. There is an emphasis on enabling young carers to fulfil their educational potential and enjoy the same opportunities as their peers. The strategy promotes a model local memorandum of understanding developed by the Associations of Directors of Adult Social Services and Directors of Children's Services (2009), and a young carer e-learning module for school staff (see http://professionals.carers.org/young-carers/articles/e-learning-for-school-staff,7023,PR.html, last accessed December 2011). The Department for Education funded Young Carer Pathfinders to develop innovative ways of identifying, assessing and supporting young carers and their families, which have since been evaluated (Department for Education 2011c).

Carers (Recognition and Services) Act 1995, Carers and Disabled Children Act 2000 and Carers (Equal Opportunities) Act 2004

Under the 1995 Act, carers are able to request an assessment of their ability to care, which should inform the local authority's decision on whether to provide services. Section 1 of the Carers and Disabled Children Act 2000 clarifies that right, specifying that carers aged 16 and over have a right to request an assessment if the person for whom they are caring is someone for whom the local authority may provide community care services. The 2004 Act ensures that any assessment must take into account the carer's employment or wish to be employed, or to take part in an education, training or leisure activity.

Disability

The Equality Act 2010 replaced most of the existing disability discrimination legislation introduced through the Disability Discrimination Acts of 1995 and 2005. In the 2010 Act, a person has a disability if: they have a physical or mental impairment; and the impairment has a substantial and long-term adverse effect on their ability to perform normal day-to-day activities. Service providers are placed under a duty to make reasonable adjustments to premises or to the way they provide a service to ensure services are accessible to disabled people, and disability is covered under the public sector equality duty which requires public bodies to eliminate unlawful discrimination and promote equality of opportunity and good relations.

References

These references are specific to this appendix. Published works cited here and in the main text are listed in the Bibliography.

Association of Directors of Adult Social Services/Association of Directors of Children's Services (2009) *Working Together to Support Young Carers.*

Department for Children, Schools and Families (2007) *Guidance on Education-Related Parenting Contracts, Parenting Orders and Penalty Notices.*

Department for Education (2011a) *The Munro Review of Child Protection Final Report: A child-centred system.*

Department for Education (2011b) *A Child-centred System. The Government's response to the Munro review of child protection.*

Department for Education (2011c) *Turning Around the Lives of Families with Multiple Problems - an evaluation of the Family and Young Carer Pathfinders Programme.*

Department for Education (2011d) *Family and Friends Care: Statutory Guidance for Local Authorities.*

Department for Education/Department of Health (2011) *Supporting families on the foundation years.*

Department of Health (2006a) *Best Practice Guidance on the role of the Director of Adult Social Services.*

Department of Health (2006b) *Guidance on the Statutory Chief Officer Post of the Director of Adult Social Services.*

Department of Health (2008) *Code of Practice Mental Health Act 1983.* London: The Stationery Office.

Department of Health (2010a) *A Vision for Adult Social Care: Capable communities and active citizens.*

Department of Health (2010b) *Prioritising Need in the Context of Putting People First: A whole system approach to eligibility for social care.*

Department of Health (2010c) *Equity and excellence: Liberating the NHS.*

Department of Health (2010d) *Healthy lives, healthy people White Paper: Our strategy for public health in England.*

Department for Work and Pensions (2010) *Universal Credit: Welfare that works.*

Gruer, L and Ainsworth, T (2003) *Hidden Harm: Responding to the needs of children of problem drug users.* London: Home Office.

HM Treasury (2010) *Spending Review 2010.* London: The Stationery Office.

HM Government (2008) *Information sharing: Guidance for practitioners and managers.*

HM Government (2010a) *Reducing Demand, Restricting Supply, Building Recovery: Supporting people to live a drug free life.*

HM Government (2010b) *Recognised, Valued and Supported: Next steps for the Carers Strategy.*

Appendix 3: Assessment practice tool

The following form was adapted by Hart and Powell (National Children's Bureau 2001, unpublished) from the Standing Conference on Drug Abuse (SCODA) guidelines for professionals assessing risk of harm to children when working with drug-using parents. The guidelines have been adapted so that the information is collated under the dimensions of the *Framework for Assessment of Children in Need and their Families* (Department of Health and others 2000).

The assessment of parents who use drugs

Assessment of family functioning and the impact it has on parental capacity

1. Pattern of parental drug use

- Is there a drug-free or supportive partner?
- Is the drug use stable or chaotic? (i.e. swings between states of intoxication and withdrawal and/or polydrug use)
- Is alcohol a part of the repertoire of drug use?
- Exactly what drugs are used? (ask specific questions, e.g. refer to yesterday or last weekend)
- How much is spent on an average day or week?
- Have there been any (voluntary) significant drug-free periods?
- What is the history of drug use? Is it escalating? Is it a response to specific events or stressful periods?
- How are the drugs used? (e.g. injected or smoked)
- What are the behavioural implications? (e.g. inconsistent behaviour, drowsiness or unavailability)

2. How the drugs are procured

- Are the children left alone while the parents are procuring drugs or getting the money to do so?
- Are the children being taken to places where they could be vulnerable?
- Where does the money to buy drugs come from?
- Are the parents frequently arrested? Are there any criminal offences still to be dealt with? Are the parents on probation?
- Is the home used for selling drugs, stolen items or prostitution?
- Are the parents allowing the home to be used by other drug users?

3. Health risks

- Where are the drugs normally kept? Could children have access to them?
- If parents are injecting drugs, are needles shared? How are syringes or needles disposed of?
- Are the parents or children registered with a GP? Is the GP aware of the drug use?

- Are the children ever given drugs?
- Do the parents have health problems associated with drug use?

4. Parents' perception of the situation

- Do the parents see their drug use as harmful to themselves or their children?
- What strategies are used to minimise the impact on the children?
- Do the parents perceive a difference in their child care when they are using drugs and when not?

5. Pregnancy

- Was drug use revealed during the pregnancy? At what stage?
- Was the mother in treatment during the pregnancy? If so, were any other drugs used in addition to those prescribed?
- At what gestation period did the mother book for antenatal care?
- If the baby needed hospital treatment for withdrawal symptoms, how did the parents cope during this time? What observations were made of their care and visiting of the baby?

Environmental factors

1. Physical needs/home environment

- Is the accommodation adequate for the children?
- Does the family move frequently?
- Are other drug users sharing the accommodation?
- Can the parents control what happens in the home?
- Is there adequate food, clothing and warmth for the children?
- Have employment and income been affected by parental drug use?

2. Social networks and support

- Do the parents and children associate mainly with other drug users?
- What support is available from extended family and friends? Do they know about the drug use?
- Are the parents in treatment now or have they been in the past? What services have helped in the past?
- Do the parents know what help and resources are available locally? What are the barriers to accessing help?

Children's developmental needs

1. Family and social relationships

- Do the children have contact with other adults outside the family? Is there a consistent, caring adult who can meet their cognitive and emotional needs?
- Do the children have age-appropriate friendships outside the home or are the family stigmatised because of drug use?

2. Emotional and behavioural development

- The older children of drug-using parents can sometimes assume inappropriate parental responsibility. Is this the case? Are they young carers themselves?
- Are the children being left to fend for themselves or look after younger siblings?

■ Consider what the children's experience of home life would be. How would they experience their parents' behaviour? Does it concern, frighten or embarrass them?

3. Health

■ Are the children registered with a GP and receiving routine health surveillance?
■ What information do the children have about substance misuse? Do they know about their parents' drug use?

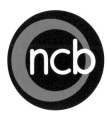

Vulnerable Children Programme

The Vulnerable Children Programme comprises NCB's practice improvement work targeting children most at risk of experiencing inequalities and poor life chances. Our focus is on those whose experience of multiple, adverse, overlapping factors in their lives make them vulnerable to significant risk of poor outcomes. Our current work is particularly concerned with the following groups of children:

- young people in the justice system
- children in care
- young people excluded from/disaffected with education
- children in need of protection
- young people living with or closely affected by HIV.

We aim:

- to use high quality research and evidence to influence policy and improve practice
- to support the development of comprehensive, holistic, responsive services providing effective and timely support for children and families
- to promote the involvement of children in shaping practices and policy to improve their lives.

We do this through running a number of discrete projects, creating and testing good quality materials and practical tools with frontline practitioners and managers, developing succinct briefings on research and policy, and providing opportunities for learning including training, action learning sets and facilitated practice exchange events for peers to learn from each other and find solutions to common problems.

For further information visit www.ncb.org.uk

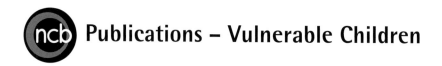

Publications – Vulnerable Children

Adult Drug Problems, Children's Needs

Assessing the impact of parental drug use
Di Hart and Jane Powell

It is widely accepted that parental problem drug use can cause serious harm to children. By working together, children's services can take practical steps to protect the children involved and improve their outlooks. With summaries of key messages, tools and tips, training and development activities, and practice examples, *Adult Drug Problems, Children's Needs* supports practitioners in their work and is aimed at all agencies that become involved with families of drug misusing parents.

2007 138pp ISBN 978 1 904787 97 6
Price £20.00 / NCB members £16.00

Milieu-therapy with children

Planned environment therapy in Scandinavia
Edited by Hans Kornerup

'The well-developed theoretical base and practice presented here helps expand our appreciation of the importance and effectiveness of Residential Child Care as 'therapy in and through the environment'.
Jonathan Stanley, Manager, NCB Residential Child Care

2009 369pp ISBN 8 788503 56 9
Price £22.99 / NCB members £17.60

My Turn to Talk

Guides to help children and young people in care to have a say about how they are looked after
Claire Lanyon and Ruth Sinclair

Updated in 2009, these illustrated guides offer practical tips for children on how they can have a say in how they are cared for. They include a description of the care planning process, advice on how to have more say in decisions about their care, what can be done if they are unhappy or have a complaint, and where to go for extra help.

2005, updated 2009 20pp each
Guide for Young People Aged 12 and Over
ISBN 1 904787 39 8
Guide for Children Aged 11 or Younger
ISBN 1 904787 40 1
Price £9.95 / NCB members £7.96

Putting Analysis into Assessment

Undertaking the assessment of needs –
a toolkit for practitioners
2nd edition
Ruth Dalzell and Emma Sawyer

Addressing issues of concern to child care social workers, particularly analytical assessment and how to avoid common pitfalls in thinking and practice, *Putting Analysis into Assessment* is the essential guide to improving assessment practice in child care social work. It provides strong theoretical foundations, and successfully demonstrates how these ideas can be translated into practice. With reference to the Framework for the Assessment of Children in Need and their Families and the Common Assessment Framework, as well as specialist assessments, the book covers every stage of the assessment process – including planning and preparation, hypothesising, involving children, making, recording and reviewing decisions.

2011 168pp ISBN 978 1 907969 29 4
Price £19.99 / NCB members £16.00

Putting Corporate Parenting into Practice

Developing an effective approach –
a toolkit for councils
Di Hart and Alison Williams

This toolkit provides practical support to those with responsibility for services for looked after children and care leavers. A CD-ROM includes a film case study of corporate parenting in action, presentations, activities, briefing papers and practice examples.

2008 128pp ISBN 978 1 905818 21 1
Price £26.00 / NCB members £20.80

Putting Corporate Parenting into Practice

Understanding the councillor's role – a handbook for councillors
Di Hart and Alison Williams

This handbook is essential reading for all local councillors and supports elected members and council officers to ensure that they effectively fulfil their role as corporate parents. It sets out the responsibilities of a corporate parent, together with practical exercises and briefings to support effective practice.

2008 76pp ISBN 978 1 905818 22 8
Price £12.00 / NCB members £9.60
Ebook £7.50 / NCB members £6.00

Reuniting Looked After Children with their Families

A review of the research
Nina Biehal

Family reunification offers a potential route to permanency for looked after children, which is a key issue in contemporary social care. This publication offers policymakers and practitioners a critical review of the research findings on family reunification available in the UK and the USA.

2006 128pp ISBN 1 904787 64 9
Price £13.95 / NCB members £11.16
Published by NCB for the Joseph Rowntree Foundation

Talking About Alcohol and Other Drugs

A guide for looked after children's services
Mary Ryan and Jo Butcher

This practice guide for corporate parents and practitioners caring for looked after children and young people provides help on developing or reviewing drug education policy and practice, and the management of drug incidents.

2006 96pp ISBN 1 904787 78 9
Price £15.00 / NCB members £12.00
Ebook £7.00 NCB members £5.60

Understanding What Children Say

Children's experiences of domestic violence, parental substance misuse and parental health problems
Sarah Gorin

The complex dynamics that can surround families dealing with issues such as domestic violence, parental substance misuse and parental health problems may make it difficult for parents and professionals to understand how children feel.
This literature review considers what children say about living in families where these issues arise. Examining research undertaken in the UK, it describes the key themes in children's experiences, how they feel about the difficulties experienced at home, what their coping strategies are and the support they would like to receive.

2004 120pp ISBN 1 904787 12 6
Price £13.95 / NCB members £11.16

Understanding Why

Understanding attachment and how this can affect education
Mary Ryan

Understanding Why describes behaviours and feelings that are common among many children and young people who have who have experienced attachment difficulties, often because of a major loss or trauma early in their lives. Written for teachers, teaching assistants, lecturers, school nurses, education support staff for looked after and vulnerable children, foster and other carers, residential child care workers, and parents of children and young people, it will help:

- teachers and others in education settings recognise attachment difficulties and consider how to help a child or young person achieve their full potential
- parents, carers and others with care responsibilities recognise attachment needs and to work together with schools to support the child or young person's successful learning.

2006 12pp ISBN: 978 1 905818 02 0
Price: £6.00 / NCB members £4.80
Ebook: £4.50 / NCB members £3.60

What Works in Residential Child Care

A review of research evidence and the practical considerations
Roger Clough, Roger Bullock, Adrian Ward

What Works in Residential Child Care reviews the state of residential child care for children and young people, highlighting what is known and the limits of knowledge, with a view to developing effective policy and practice. Using residential services in Wales as its case study, the key messages of the book apply throughout the UK. It includes a literature review that draws on research in the UK and the US.

2006 134pp ISBN: 1 904787 77 0
Price: £12.00 / NCB members £9.60
Ebook: £7.00 / NCB members £5.60

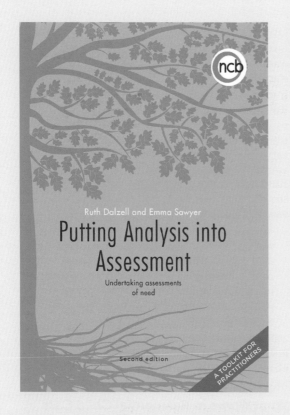

Putting Analysis into Assessment

Undertaking the assessment of needs –
a toolkit for practitioners
2nd edition
Ruth Dalzell and Emma Sawyer

*'As social workers are striving to push back the
excessive levels of bureaucratisation and increase
the space for professional practice, this excellent
book offers easily understood ways to improve
critical reasoning skills and will be useful for
individuals, teams, and agencies.'*

Professor Eileen Munro
Social Policy Department,
London School of Economics

Addressing issues of concern to child care social workers, particularly analytical assessment and how to
avoid common pitfalls in thinking and practice, *Putting Analysis into Assessment* is the essential guide
to improving assessment practice in child care social work. It provides strong theoretical foundations,
and successfully demonstrates how these ideas can be translated into practice.

With reference to the Framework for the Assessment of Children in Need and their Families and the
Common Assessment Framework, as well as specialist assessments, the book covers every stage of the
assessment process – including planning and preparation, hypothesising, involving children, making,
recording and reviewing decisions.

This revised edition offers a range of new and tested practice tools, case studies, practice development
sessions and activities, plus new sections on risk and resilience and assessing need and risk in chronic
situations. The toolkit will:

- aid practitioners in their thinking before, during and at the conclusion of their work with children
  and families
- provide managers with materials to use in supervision and team development
- enable trainers to deliver training to those involved in social work and interagency assessments
- offer lecturers practical tools and stimulating materials that will help students bridge the worlds
  of theory and practice.

2011 168pp ISBN 978 1 907969 29 4
Price £19.99 / NCB members £16.00

NCB Membership

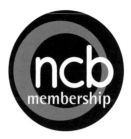

NCB is the largest multi-agency membership network for children's services and studies in the country.

With nearly 50 years experience of working across the children's sector, developing best practice and sharing expertise between agencies, NCB is the place to go for information that cuts through the spin and gets straight to the facts.

Stay informed
Specialist bulletins, digests and briefings.

Get involved
Contribute to our strategic direction and share in best practice discussion.

Save money
Discounted publications, subscriptions, events and journals.

Join today for exclusive and practical benefits, discounts and support services:

www.ncb.org.uk/join

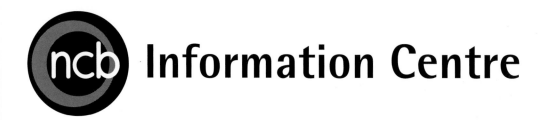 **Information Centre**

The largest collection of resources about children and young people's issues in the UK.

NCB's Information Centre and Library has a comprehensive and multi-disciplinary collection of books, journals and grey literature on all aspects of children and young people's social care, health and education.

The collection contains over 30,000 publications and 250 British and international journal titles. Most of the resources in the collection are published in the UK but we do also have European and international material. We have a large statistical collection and aim to collect all government legislation relating to children and young people.

Information Centre Access

The Information Centre is open to visitors from 10am to 5pm, Monday to Friday.
Access is free for NCB Members.
The rate for non-members is £10 per day.
To make an appointment, please call us on +44 (0)20 7843 6008.

Enquiries

Phone: +44 (0)20 7843 6008
Email: library@ncb.org.uk
Address: Information Centre
National Children's Bureau
8 Wakley Street, London EC1V 7QE